Study Guide

to accompany

Whaley & Wong's
Nursing Care of Infants and Children

Fifth Edition

Anne Rath Rentfro, MSN, RN, CS, CDE
Assistant Professor of Nursing,
The University of Texas at Brownsville
in Partnership with Texas Southmost College,
Brownsville, Texas

Linda S. McCampbell, MSN, RN, CS, FNP
Assistant Professor of Nursing,
The University of Texas at Brownsville
in Partnership with Texas Southmost College,
Brownsville, Texas;
Family Nurse Practitioner,
Rio Hondo Health Clinic,
Rio Hondo, Texas

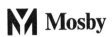 Mosby

St. Louis Baltimore Boston Carlsbad Chicago Naples New York Philadelphia Portland
London Madrid Mexico City Singapore Sydney Tokyo Toronto Wiesbaden

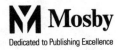

Mosby
Dedicated to Publishing Excellence

**A Times Mirror
Company**

Publisher: Nancy L. Coon
Senior Editor: Sally Schrefer
Developmental Editor: Janet R. Livingston
Manuscript Editor: Susan Warrington
Design and Layout: Ken Wendling

Printed in the United States of America
Composition by Wordbench
Printing/binding by Plus Communications

Mosby-Year Book, Inc.
11830 Westline Industrial Drive
St. Louis, Missouri 63146

International Standard Book Number 0-8151-9395-5

95 96 97 98 99 / 9 8 7 6 5 4 3 2 1

Contributor

Elisabeth Boone
St. Louis, Missouri
Chapters 1-40: Crossword Puzzles

Preface

This Study Guide accompanies the fifth edition of *Whaley & Wong's Nursing Care of Infants and Children*. Students may use the Study Guide not only to review content but also to enhance their learning through critical thinking. The Study Guide's purpose is to assist students in mastering the content presented in the text, developing problem-solving skills, and applying their knowledge to nursing practice.

The Study Guide includes questions that will assist the student to meet the objectives of each corresponding textbook chapter. Because most students using this Study Guide will also be preparing to pass the nursing examination (NCLEX), we have chosen a multiple-choice format. A Critical Thinking section is included for each chapter. The questions in the Critical Thinking section help students analyze the chapter's content and address their own attitudes about pediatric nursing practice. Case Studies were used in many of the Critical Thinking sections to help students address specific practice issues. All case presentations are fictitious but designed to address situations that are frequently encountered by the nurse in practice. Crossword puzzles are included to help students learn and retain new terminology and commonly used abbreviations that are used in each chapter.

How to Use the Study Guide

We intend for the student to use this Study Guide while he or she studies a chapter in the textbook, processing the material chapter by chapter and section by section. For this reason we chose to present the questions in an order that follows the textbook's content. The student may find the answers to the questions by using the page number references provided for each chapter at the end of the Study Guide. This format was chosen so that the student refers back to the textbook to find the answer, rather than checking his or her answer against an answer key.

The Instructor's Resource Kit that accompanies the fifth edition of *Whaley & Wong's Nursing Care of Infants and Children* contains the specific answers for the questions. This allows the instructor the option of assigning questions from the Study Guide as structured homework.

It is our hope that this Study Guide will function as both an aid to learning and a means for measuring progress in the mastery of pediatric nursing practice.

Anne R. Rentfro
Linda S. McCampbell

Contents

❖ CHAPTER 1
Perspectives of Pediatric Nursing

1. Which one of the following objectives would NOT be considered a "Healthy People 2000" priority area for the 1990s?
   A. improve nutritional and infant health
   B. eradicate acute respiratory disorders in infants
   C. reduce violent and abusive behavior
   D. expand community-based health promotion programs

2. Which one of the following statements is TRUE about infant mortality in the United States?
   A. Infant mortality is at an all-time high in the U.S.
   B. The U.S. currently holds its lowest infant mortality rate ever.
   C. Infant mortality rates in the U.S. are higher than in other developed countries.
   D. The U.S. has a lower mortality rate than Canada.

3. Which one of the following risks for neonatal mortality increased in 1991 and is considered a key factor in the higher U.S. neonatal mortality rates when compared with other countries?
   A. birth weight less than 2500 grams
   B. short or long gestational age
   C. race and gender
   D. lower level of maternal education

4. Which one of the following accounts for more than 20% of the deaths in infants under 1 year of age?
   A. pneumonia and influenza
   B. infections specific to the perinatal period
   C. accidents and adverse effects
   D. congenital anomalies

5. Neural tube defects are expected to decrease by as much as 50% with the current recommendation by the American

   Academy of Pediatrics for all women of childbearing age to receive _____ _____ supplementation.

6. Which one of the following differences is seen when infant death rates are categorized according to race? Infant mortality for:
   A. Native Americans has decreased due to post neonatal mortality.
   B. Hispanics may not include all Hispanic subgroups.
   C. blacks is five times the rate for whites.
   D. whites is the same as for other races.

7. After a child reaches the age of 1, the leading cause of death is from:
   A. violent deaths.
   B. congenital anomalies.
   C. cancer.
   D. injuries.

8. Which two diseases are becoming more prominent on the list of leading causes of death during childhood?
   A. neoplasm and tuberculosis
   B. tuberculosis and acquired immunodeficiency syndrome (AIDS)
   C. neoplasm and AIDS
   D. infectious diseases and AIDS

9. Morbidity statistics which depict the prevalence of a specific illness in the population are:
   A. presented as rates per 100 population.
   B. difficult to define.
   C. denoting acute illness only.
   D. denoting chronic disease only.

10. Fifty percent of all acute conditions of childhood can be accounted for by:
    A. injuries and accidents.
    B. bacterial infections.
    C. parasitic disease.
    D. respiratory illness.

11. The degree of disability can be measured by:
    A. days of hospitalization.
    B. developmental stages.
    C. days off from school or confined to bed.
    D. physical growth patterns.

12. Identify one major category of disease that children tend to contract in infancy and early childhood.

    _____

13. List three factors that contribute to increasing the morbidity of any disorder in children.

    _____

    _____

    _____

14. Another term for the *new morbidity* is:
    A. pediatric social illness.
    B. pediatric noncompliance.
    C. learning disorder.
    D. dyslexia.

15. Which one of the following statements about injuries in childhood is FALSE?
    A. Developmental stage determines the prevalence of injuries at a given age.
    B. Most fatal injuries occur in children under the age of nine.
    C. Developmental stage helps to direct preventive measures.
    D. The highest incidence of injury occurs in children under the age of 9.

16. Identify the following strategies as either *passive* or *active* prevention measures.

    _____ A. childproof medicine caps

    _____ B. airbags

    _____ C. smoke detectors

_____ D. seat belts

_____ E. safety restraints

_____ F. automatic seat belts

_____ G. warning labels

_____ H. automatic fire sprinklers

_____ I. education about firearms

_____ J. anticipatory guidance

_____ K. window guards

_____ L. mandatory seat belt laws

_____ M. bicycle helmet laws

_____ N. childproof cigarette lighters

_____ O. swimming pool fences

_____ P. swimming pool surface alarm

17. Which one of the following statements about injury prevention in children is TRUE?
    A. Including only the mother may be the most effective teaching strategy with the Hispanic population.
    B. Less than 30% of pediatric nurse practitioners routinely give advice about child car restraints.
    C. Most pediatric nurse practitioners routinely give advice about child car restraints.
    D. Parents are usually aware of their child's developmental progress and capabilities.

18. _____ _____ is the term used for teaching and counseling of parents and others about developmental expectations that serves to alert the parents to the issues that are most likely to arise at a given age.

19. Child health care in the United States has evolved from the colonial era, with its many hazards and epidemics, to the advances of the twentieth century when studies of economic and social factors stimulated the creation of better standards of care for mothers and children. Indicate whether each statement better reflects _colonial_ times or modern (_industrial_) times.

_____ nurses needing to be aware of economics

_____ milk stations

_____ illiterate parents

_____ knowledge barriers (such as not knowing about available services)

_____ rooming in, sibling visitation, child life (play) programs

_____ scarcity of books

_____ the dawn of improved health care

_____ Maternal and Child Health, Crippled Children's Services, and child welfare services

_____ Quackery is common.

_____ Lina Rogers became the first full-time school nurse.

_____ decline in infant mortality

_____ Exposure to new fatal diseases is common.

_____ prevention and health promotion measures

_____ Lillian Wald founded the Henry St. Settlement.

_____ Spitz and Robertson demonstrated the effects of isolation and maternal deprivation

_____ statistics on childhood mortality unavailable

_____ Parents were prohibited from visiting sick children.

_____ isolation and maternal deprivation

_____ training based on past experiences

_____ Lillian Wald, the founder of community nursing

_____ parent education

_____ hospital schooling

_____ epidemic diseases

_____ cow's milk as the chief source of bovine tuberculosis

_____ financial barriers such as not having insurance

_____ smallpox, measles, mumps, chickenpox, and influenza

_____ School health helped to develop pediatric courses.

_____ diagnosis related groups (DRGs)

_____ diphtheria, yellow fever, cholera, and whooping cough

_____ cow's milk as the chief source of infantile diarrhea

_____ Nurses were employed to teach parents and children.

_____ prehospitalization preparation

_____ dysentery

_____ Abraham Jacobi, the Father of Pediatrics

_____ unknown control for diseases

_____ sanitation and pasteurization of cow's milk

_____ system barriers such as state-to-state variations

_____ American Medical Association opposes the Maternity and Infancy Act.

_____ American Academy of Pediatrics is created.

_____ medical care limited to the wealthy

_____ Title V of the Social Security Act passes.

_____ physician shortage

_____ the White House Conference on Children

20. Match the federal program with the impact it has on maternal and child health.

A. Education of the Handicapped Act Amendments of 1986 (P.L. 99-457)

B. Social Services Block Grant

C. Alcohol, Drug Abuse, and Mental Health Block Grants

D. Education for All Handicapped Children Act (P.L. 94-1432)

E. Medicaid

F. Family and Medical Leave Act (FMLA)

G. Aid to Families with Dependent Children (AFDC)

H. MCH Service Block Grant

I. Women, Infants, and Children (WIC)

_____ Created in 1965, this is the largest maternal-child health program. The Child Health Assessment Program (CHAP) provides services for children and pregnant women and children under this program. Eligibility varies from state to state.

_____ created in 1935 as a cash grant to aid needy children without fathers

_____ provides services to reduce infant mortality, disease, and handicaps and to increase access to care

_____ established in 1981 to fund projects related to substance abuse and to treat mentally disturbed children

_____ provides funds for child protective services, family planning, and foster care

_____ started in 1974 to provide nutritious food and education to low-income childbearing women, infants, and children up to age 5 years

_____ passed in 1975 to provide free public education to handicapped children

_____ provides funding for multidisciplinary programs for handicapped infants and toddlers

_____ allows employees to take unpaid leave (1993)

21. Two basic concepts in the philosophy of family-centered pediatric nursing care are:
A. enabling and empowerment.
B. empowerment and bias.
C. enabling and curing.
D. empowerment and self-control.

22. An example of atraumatic care would be to:
    A. eliminate all traumatic procedures.
    B. restrict visiting hours to adults only.
    C. perform invasive procedures only in the treatment room.
    D. permit traditional clinical practices.

23. A care delivery system that balances quality and cost and that has been shown to improve satisfaction, decrease fragmentation, and measure patient outcomes would best describe:
    A. case management.
    B. primary nursing.
    C. family-centered nursing.
    D. functional nursing.

24. Match the role of the pediatric nurse with its description.

    A. family advocacy/caring   _____ a mutual exchange of ideas and opinions

    B. disease prevention/ health promotion   _____ extending to include the community or society as a whole

    C. health teaching   _____ health maintenance strategies

    D. support   _____ working together as a member of the health team

    E. counseling   _____ providing physical and emotional care (feeding/bathing)

    F. restorative care   _____ systematically recording and analyzing observations

    G. coordination/collaboration   _____ attention to emotional needs (listening/physical presence)

    H. ethical decision making   _____ transmitting information

    I. research   _____ using patient/family/societal values in care

    J. health care planning   _____ acting in the child's best interest

❖ Critical Thinking ❖
Case Study

Marisa Gutierrez arrives with her infant, Sara, at the Well Baby Clinic. Sara, who is 14 months old, is the youngest of three children. Her mother has brought her to the clinic for well child care.

Sara's two brothers, who are 7 and 8 years old, have come along. As you are interviewing her mother, Sara explores the examination room. She reaches for her older brother's marbles and puts one in her mouth.

25. After organizing the data into similar categories, the nurse makes which one of the following decisions?
    A. No dysfunctional health problems are evident.
    B. High risk for dysfunctional health problems exists.
    C. Actual dysfunctional health problems are evident.
    D. Potential complications are evident.

26. The nurse then identifies a possible human response pattern to further classify the data. Which one of the following functional health patterns would be BEST for the nurse to select?
    A. Role-Relationship Pattern
    B. Nutritional-Metabolic Pattern
    C. Coping-Stress Tolerance Pattern
    D. Self-Perception—Self-Concept Pattern

27. Based on the data collected, which one of the following nursing diagnoses would be MOST appropriate?
    A. altered family processes
    B. ineffective family coping
    C. ineffective individual coping
    D. altered parenting

28. Which one of the following patient outcomes is individualized for Sara?
    A. Sara will receive her immunizations on time.
    B. Sara will demonstrate adherence to the nurse's recommendations.
    C. Marisa Gutierrez will verbalize the need to keep small objects away from Sara to avoid aspiration.
    D. Sara's brothers will verbalize the need to discontinue playing with small objects.

29. During the evaluation phase, which one of the following responses by Sara's mother would indicate that the expected outcomes have been met?
    A. "I will have to go through all of the boys' things when we get home to be sure there aren't any other small objects that could hurt Sara."
    B. "I had forgotten how curious babies are. It has been many years since the boys were babies, and they didn't have an older child's toys around."
    C. "I will have to start to discipline Sara now so that she knows not to play with the older children's belongings."
    D. "I am afraid she cannot receive her immunizations. She had a fever after her last one."

30. At Sara's next well baby visit, what information would be MOST important to document in the chart?
    A. written evidence of progress toward outcomes
    B. the standard care plan
    C. broad-based goals
    D. interventions applicable to patients like Sara

❖ *Crossword Puzzle* ❖

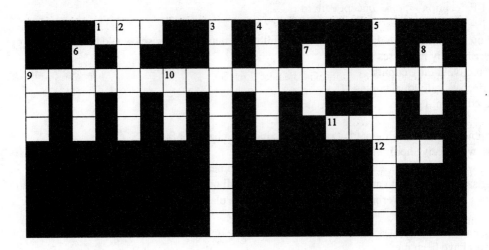

Across

1. Clinical nurse specialist
9. The number of deaths per 1000 live births during the first year of life (3 words)
11. Social Security Act
12. Low birth weight

Down

2. North American Nursing Diagnosis Association
3. Illness
4. Joint Commission on Accreditation of Healthcare Organizations
5. Death
6. Aid to Families with Dependent Children
7. Woman, Infants, and Children
8. All-terrain vehicle
9. International Classification of Diseases
10. Maternal-child health

❖ CHAPTER 2
Social, Cultural, and Religious Influences on Child Health Promotion

1. When considering the impact of culture on the pediatric client, the nurse recognizes that culture:
   A. is synonymous with race.
   B. affects the development of health beliefs.
   C. refers to a group of people with similar physical characteristics.
   D. refers to the universal manner and sequence of growth and development.

2. Which of the following social groups is an example of a primary group?
   A. six inseparable teenagers
   B. a second-grade class
   C. the members of a national church
   D. the city garden club

3. The use of guilt and shame by a culture provides:
   A. feelings of comfort about wrongdoing.
   B. an outlet following wrongdoing.
   C. rewards for culturally acceptable social behavior.
   D. internalization of the cultural norms.

4. Match the subcultural influence with the phrase or sentence that describes the word or its influence on a child's cultural development.

A. ethnicity	_____	Purchased surrogates may provide the adult authority.
B. ethnocentrism	_____	Language is often a major educational controversy.
C. social class	_____	lack of resources needed for adequate shelter
D. poverty	_____	After family, this has the most impact on a child's socialization.
E. homelessness	_____	differentiation is based on distinguishing factors such as customs
F. migrant families	_____	limit of resources needed for adequate existence
G. affluence	_____	belief that one's own ethnic group is superior to others
H. religion	_____	lack of continuity in education and health care
I. school	_____	dictates the code of morality
J. peers	_____	synonymous with occupation in the United States
K. biculture	_____	increase in influence as child moves through school

5. Currently in North America there is less reliance on tradition, families are fragmented, and transmission of customs is limited because of:
   A. a growing proportion of ethnic minorities.
   B. more emphasis on ethnic diversity.
   C. the frontier background of the American culture.
   D. increasing geographic and economic mobility.

6. Which country has more racial, ethnic, and religious minority groups than any other country?
   A. United States
   B. Mexico
   C. Canada
   D. India

7. Which of the following groups is the largest minority group in the United States?
   A. Spanish/Hispanic
   B. black
   C. Asian
   D. Latino

8. The term *Latino* refers to individuals:
   A. who are Mexican-American, Cuban, and Colombian.
   B. with a Spanish surname.
   C. from Mexico and Central America.
   D. from the Spanish-speaking countries.

9. A child has become acculturated when:
   A. a gradual process of ethnic blending occurs.
   B. the child identifies with traditional heritage.
   C. ethnic and racial pride emerge.
   D. counteraggressive behavior is eliminated.

10. Which of the following strategies would be likely to produce the most conflict when considering the concept of cultural shock?
    A. teaching the family some of the dominant culture's customs
    B. using the child to translate for the parent
    C. identifying some of the usual family customs
    D. learning tolerance of other's values and beliefs

11. Cultural beliefs and practices are an important part of nursing assessment, because when analyzed and incorporated into the nursing process, beliefs:
    A. may sometimes expedite the plan of care.
    B. can be manipulated more easily if known.
    C. must be in unison with standard health practices.
    D. are very similar from one culture to another.

12. An innate susceptibility is acquired through:
    A. the child's general physical status.
    B. exposure to environmental factors.
    C. long-term proximity to disease.
    D. generations of evolutionary changes.

13. Match the racial/ethnic group with its commonly associated disease.

A. Tay-Sachs disease _____ Greek

B. cystic fibrosis _____ Middle Eastern

C. sickle cell disease _____ Japanese

D. neural tube defects _____ Jewish

E. cleft lip/palate _____ Irish

F. beta-thalassemia _____ Polynesian

G. clubfoot _____ Navaho Indian

H. ear anomalies _____ African black

I. Werdnig-Hoffmann disease _____ English/Scottish

14. In which of the following ethnic groups would the finding of phenylketonuria be considered unusual?
A. Scandinavian
B. Scottish/Irish
C. Mediterranean
D. Middle Eastern

15. Lactose intolerance symptoms usually become problematic at around the age of:
A. 1 to 3 years.
B. 3 to 5 years.
C. 1 to 3 months.
D. 3 to 5 months.

16. Sickle cell anemia is an example of selective advantage against which of the following diseases?
A. phenylketonuria
B. diphtheria
C. tuberculosis
D. malaria

17. When considering social, cultural, and religious factors in a child's development, the nurse recognizes that the MOST overwhelming influence on health is the individual's:
A. genetic background.
B. proximity to the disease.
C. socioeconomic status.
D. health beliefs and practices.

18. The concept that any behavior must be judged first in relation to the context of the culture in which it occurs is called:
A. cultural relativity.
B. cultural stereotyping.
C. nonverbal communication.
D. culturally sensitive interaction.

19. Match the custom with the ethnic group.

A. Jewish   _____   Eye contact may be considered a sign of hostility.

B. United States (dominant culture)   _____   Nonverbal communication is a practiced art.

C. Hispanic   _____   seek to avoid disharmony

D. Oriental   _____   focus on time and use the expression "time flies"

E. American Indian   _____   believe that the male child will take care of his parents in their old age

F. Asian   _____   believe that infants can develop symptoms of the "evil eye"

20. Which of the following strategies would NOT be considered culturally sensitive?
    A. active listening
    B. slow and careful speaking
    C. loud and clear speaking
    D. repetition and clarification

21. Which of the following groups of food would be common to most cultures?
    A. chicken, tomatoes, rice, apples
    B. pork, broccoli, noodles, bananas
    C. sausage, carrots, dry cereal, oranges
    D. beef, green beans, oatmeal, pears

22. Match the food with the ethnic group that food is associated with.

A. black   _____   curry

B. Hispanic   _____   raw tuna

C. Japanese   _____   lychee

D. Chinese   _____   nopales

E. Vietnamese   _____   bok choy

F. Eastern Indian   _____   chitterlings

23. All of the following factors have been shown to affect food preferences and traditions EXCEPT:
    A. age.
    B. availability.
    C. religion.
    D. gender.

24. Voodoo is an example of an influence that would be considered:
    A. a supernatural force.
    B. a natural force.
    C. an imbalance of the forces.
    D. an imbalance of the four humors.

25. Adopting a multicultural perspective means that the nurse:
    A. explains that biomedical measures are usually more effective.
    B. uses the client's traditional health and cultural beliefs.
    C. realizes that most folk remedies have a scientific basis.
    D. uses aspects of the cultural beliefs to develop a plan.

26. Which of the following terms is NOT used to describe a kind of folk healer?
    A. asafetida
    B. curandera
    C. curandero
    D. kahuna

27. Which of the following health practices may compromise the health and well-being of either mother or fetus?
    A. the mother reaching her arms above her head
    B. the practice of eating azarcon
    C. the use of asafetida
    D. the practice of ho'oponopono

28. To provide culturally sensitive care to children and their families, the nurse should:
    A. disregard his/her own cultural values.
    B. identify behavior that is abnormal.
    C. recognize characteristic behaviors of certain cultures.
    D. rely on own feelings and experiences for guidance.

29. In planning and implementing transcultural patient care, nurses need to strive to:
    A. adapt the family's ethnic practices to the health need.
    B. change the family's long-standing beliefs.
    C. use traditional ethnic practices in every client's care.
    D. teach the family only how to treat the health problem.

30. Generalizations about cultural groups are important for nurses to know, because this information helps the nurse to:
    A. learn the similarities among all cultures.
    B. learn the unique practices of various groups.
    C. stereotype groups' characteristics.
    D. categorize groups according to their similarities.

❖ Critical Thinking ❖

31. During assessment a client reveals that her family uses an acupuncturist occasionally. Based on this information, the nurse would realize that another health practice commonly found in the same cultural group would be:
    A. voodoo.
    B. moxibustion.
    C. santeria.
    D. kampo.

32. Cultural assessment data would be MOST important for which of the following nursing diagnoses?
    A. decreased cardiac output
    B. impaired skin integrity
    C. ineffective airway clearance
    D. altered nutrition

33. In planning any food list for the client whose family holds beliefs of the Black Muslims, which of the following foods would be the MOST appropriate to include?

    A. pork
    B. corn bread
    C. rice
    D. collard greens

34. Using a framework to evaluate transcultural nursing care, the nurse would identify which of the following health practices as typical?

    A. A Japanese family cares for a disabled family member in their home.
    B. An American black family uses amulets as a shield from witchcraft.
    C. A Puerto Rican family seeks help from a curandera.
    D. A Mexican-American family seeks help from santeros.

❖ Crossword Puzzle ❖

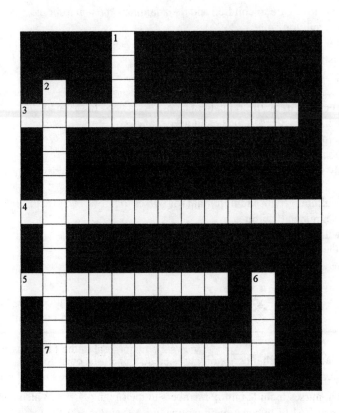

Across

3. Labeling and lack of recognition of differences among people within a particular cultural, ethnic, or religious group
4. Gradual changes produced in a culture by the influence of another culture
5. Shared racial, cultural, social, and linguistic heritage
7. Smaller group within a culture

Down

1. Expected behavior of individuals in a particular culture
2. Emotional attitude that one's own ethnic group is superior to other ethnic groups
6. Group of people with similar physical characteristics

❖ CHAPTER 3
Family Influences on Child Health Promotion

1. Which one of the following descriptions would NOT be correct in defining the term *family* as it is viewed today?
   A. The family is what the client considers it to be.
   B. The family may be related or unrelated.
   C. The family is always related by legal ties or genetic relationships and live in the same household.
   D. The family members share a sense of belonging to their own family.

2. Match the family theory with its description. (Some theories may be used more than once.)

   A. Family Systems theory

   _____ employs crisis intervention strategies with the focus on helping members cope with challenging events

   B. Family Stress theory

   _____ continual interaction between family members and the environment

   C. Developmental theory

   _____ A problem or dysfunction is not viewed as lying in any one family member but rather in the interactions used by the family; focus is on interactions of members rather than on an individual member.

   D. Structural-Functional theory

   _____ uses concepts of basic attributes, resources, perception, and coping behaviors or strategies in assessing family crisis management

   _____ addresses family change over time based on the predictable changes in the structure, function, and roles of the family, with the age of the oldest child as the marker for stage transition

   _____ Both the family and each individual member must achieve developmental tasks as part of each family life cycle stage.

   _____ views the major goal of the family as socialization of its members into society

3. In working with children, nurses include family members in their plan of care. Which one of the following statements does the nurse recognize as FALSE when planning nursing interventions for the family?
   A. A complete family assessment is needed to discover family dynamics, family strengths, and family weaknesses.
   B. Recognition of situations where referral of the family to specialized services is needed is not a nursing responsibility.
   C. The intervention used with families will depend on the nurse's view of the theoretic model of the family.
   D. The level of assistance a family needs will depend on the type of crisis, factors affecting family adjustment, and the family's level of functioning.

4. Debbie is 2 years old and lives with her brother, Mark, her sister, Mary, and her mother. Her father and mother recently divorced and now her father lives one hour away. Debbie sees her father once a month for a day's visit. Her mother retains custody of Debbie. Debbie's grandparents live in a different state but she visits them each year. Debbie's family represents which one of the following?
   A. Binuclear Family
   B. Extended Family
   C. Single-Parent Family
   D. Reconstituted Family

5. Which one of the following is an effective approach for working with vulnerable families?
   A. Identify and emphasize family deficits.
   B. Offer single-purpose services with responses aimed at solving emergencies.
   C. Emphasize and focus on the troubled individual child or family member.
   D. Identify cultural differences, treating families with respect and honoring their traditions.

6. Identify the following statements as either TRUE or FALSE.

   _____ Roles are learned through the socialization process.

   _____ Role continuity is described as role behavior that is expected of children conflicting with desirable adult behavior.

   _____ All families have strengths and vulnerabilities.

   _____ Each family has its own standards for interaction within and outside the family.

   _____ Role definitions are changing as a result of the changing economy and the women's movement. Marital roles, however, are still most segregated among the middle classes.

7. Identify the type of role that is related to fantasy and important in childhood as a means of adjustment and socialization. In this role, the child uses the environment as a primary resource for learning the conduct that befits position or status.
   A. ascribed roles
   B. achieved roles
   C. adopted roles
   D. assumed roles

8. Children learn role behavior and to perform in expected ways within the family at a very early age. One influence of

   the role each sibling is assigned within the family structure is the _____ _____.

9. Parenting practices differ between small and large families. Which one of the following characteristics is NOT found in small families?
   A. Emphasis is placed on the individual development of the child, with constant pressure to measure up to family expectations.
   B. Adolescents identify more strongly with their parents and rely more on their parents for advice.
   C. Emphasis is placed on the group and less on the individual.
   D. Children's development and achievement are measured against children in the neighborhood and social class.

10. Because age differences between siblings affect the childhood environment, the nurse recognizes that there is more affection and less rivalry and hostility between children that are spaced how many years apart?
    A. 4 or more years
    B. 4 or fewer years
    C. 3 or fewer years
    D. 2 or fewer years

11. Johnnie has always been viewed by his parents as being less dependent than his brother, Tommy, or his sister, Julie. Johnnie is described as affectionate, good-natured, and flexible in his thinking. He identifies with his peer group and is very popular with classmates. His parents tend to place fewer demands on Johnnie for household help. From this description, the nurse would expect Johnnie to have what birth position within the family?
    A. firstborn child
    B. middle child
    C. youngest child
    D. any of the above; birth position does not affect personality

12. Monozygotic twins are:
    A. the result of fertilization of two ova.
    B. the result of fertilization of one ovum that became separated early in development.
    C. different physically and genetically.
    D. of dissimilar behaviors with greater sibling rivalry.

13. The MOST essential component of successful parenting is which one of the following?
    A. strong religious and cultural ties to the community
    B. previous experience with childcare, usually during adolescence as an older sibling or babysitter
    C. an understanding of childhood growth and development
    D. one person responsible for providing childcare within the family structure

14. Which one of the following does NOT identify a method to promote separation-individuation between twins?
    A. Parents discipline and praise twins as a unit.
    B. Parents foster feeling of separateness between twins.
    C. Parents avoid the term "the twins."
    D. Parents foster opportunities to build one-to-one relationships with each twin.

15. Development of a parental sense can be divided into four phases. Briefly describe each phase.

    A. Anticipation: _____

    B. Honeymoon: _____

    C. Plateau: _____

    D. Disengagement: _____

16. The parenting behavior of warmth-hostility is BEST described by which one of the following?
    A. the degree of autonomy that parents allow their children
    B. the degree of open or frequent parental affection combined with the degree of affection mixed with feelings of rejection or hostility that is expressed by the parents to their children
    C. the degree of restrictive control the parents impose on their children combined with the degree of active survey of their children's behavior
    D. the degree to which the parents allow their children to openly display feelings of rejection and hostility combined with the acceptance of this behavior

17. Match the parenting style with its description.

    A. authoritarian/dictatorial _____ allows children to regulate their own activity; sees the parenting role as being a resource rather than a role model

    B. permissive/laissez-faire _____ establishes rules, regulations, and standards of conduct for the child that are to be followed without question

    C. authoritative/democratic _____ respects the child's individuality; directs the child's behavior by emphasizing the reason for rules

18. Child misbehavior requires parental implementation of appropriate disciplinary action. Identify which one of the following would NOT be a correct guideline for implementing discipline.
    A. Focus on child and misbehavior, utilizing "you" messages rather than "I" messages.
    B. Maintain consistency with disciplinary action.
    C. Make sure all caregivers maintain unity of plan by agreeing on plan and being familiar with details before implementation.
    D. Maintain flexibility by planning disciplinary actions appropriate to child's age, temperament, and severity of misbehavior.

19. Which one of the following is a correct interpretation in the use of reasoning as a form of discipline?
    A. used for older children when moral issues are involved
    B. used for younger children to "see the other side" of an issue
    C. used only in combination with scolding and criticism
    D. used to allow children to obtain lengthy explanations and a greater degree of attention from parents

20. Which one of the following is NOT a description of the discipline "time out"?
    A. allows the reinforcer to be maintained
    B. no physical punishment is involved
    C. offers both parents and child "cooling off" time
    D. facilitates the parent's ability to consistently apply the punishment

21. Areas of concern for parents of adoptive children include:
    A. the initial attachment process.
    B. telling the children that they are adopted.
    C. identity formation of children during adolescence.
    D. all of the above.

22. Identify the following statements about the impact of divorce on children as either TRUE or FALSE.

    _____ Research has shown that children of divorce suffer no lasting psychologic and social difficulties.

    _____ One outcome found in children of divorce is a heightened anxiety about forming enduring relationships as young adults.

    _____ Children of divorce cope better with their feelings of abandonment when there is continuing conflict between parents.

    _____ Preschoolers assume themselves to be the cause of the divorce and interpret the separation as punishment.

    _____ School-age children's teachers and school counselors should be informed because these children will often display altered behaviors.

    _____ Adolescents have concerns and heightened anxiety about their own future as a marital partner and the availability of money for future needs.

23. Which one of the following is NOT considered important by parents when telling their children about the decision to divorce?
    A. Initial disclosure should include both parents and siblings.
    B. Time should be allowed for discussion with each child individually.
    C. The initial disclosure should be kept simple and reasons for divorce should not be included.
    D. Parents should physically hold or touch their child to provide feelings of warmth and reassurance.

24. Single-parenting, step-parenting, and dual-earner family parenting add stress to the parental role. Match the family type with an expected stressor or concern.

A. single-parenting   _____   Managing shortages of money, time, and energy are major concerns.

B. step-parenting   _____   Overload is a common source of stress, and social activities are significantly curtailed with time demands and scheduling seen as major problems.

C. dual-earner families

       _____   Competition is a major area of concern among adults, with reduction of power conflicts a necessity.

❖ Critical Thinking ❖
Case Study

Ester and Roberto Garcia are the proud new parents of twin boys, Timothy and Thomas. Ester and Roberto Garcia have been married less than one year. Ester is 17 years old and plans to return to finish school next year. Roberto finished high school and works with his father in a local auto repair shop. He is taking a week off from work to help Ester at home with Timothy and Thomas. Neither of the couple attended child parenting classes. You are making a home visit to the couple one day after they have brought Timothy and Thomas home from the hospital. As you arrive at the house you see that both Timothy and Thomas are crying. Ester is trying to give Timothy his bath while Roberto is busy trying to get Thomas to take his formula. Both new parents appear tired, and Roberto admits that they have been up all night with the infants and that either Timothy or Thomas seems to be crying "all the time" and "something must be terribly wrong with them."

25. As you begin your assessment of the family, you know that the Garcia family are in stage II, families with infants, according to Duvall's developmental stages of the family. Which one of the following is a developmental task of this stage?
A. Reestablish couple identity.
B. Socialize children.
C. Make decisions regarding parenthood.
D. Accommodate to parenting role.

26. A priority nursing diagnosis for this family would be:
A. altered family processes related to gain of family members.
B. altered growth and development related to inadequate caretaking.
C. fear related to new parental role.
D. high risk for injury related to unsafe environment.

27. As the nurse developing the plan for this new family, your priority intervention would be which one of the following?
A. teaching the parents about Duvall's developmental stages so that they will understand that what they are experiencing is normal transition into parenthood
B. reassuring the parents that you will examine each of the infants but that they appear to be healthy and that the parents are doing a good job
C. taking over the feeding and bathing of the infants, explaining to the parents the necessity of child parenting classes
D. checking the infant supplies and environment to make sure the home has been made safe for children

28. Both Thomas and Timothy are now sleeping, and you have completed your family assessment with Roberto and Ester Garcia. As a nurse you decide to use the family stress theory to promote adaptation to the family's new role. Which one of the following does the nurse know is NOT a capability the family can use to manage the crisis?
A. basic attributes of the family
B. resources within the family
C. perception of family to the situation
D. closed boundary within the family system

❖ Crossword Puzzle ❖

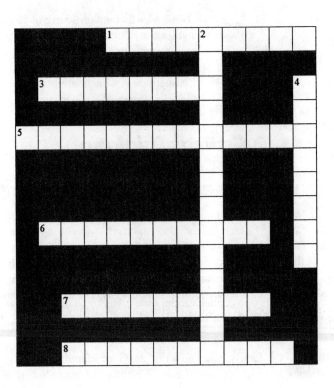

Across

1. Composition of the family
3. Establishment of a legal relationship of parent and child between persons not related by birth
5. Parental style of control in which parents make strict rules and rigidly enforce behavior
6. One or both married adults have children from a previous marriage residing in the household
7. Persons sharing a common dwelling
8. Parental style of control that allows children to regulate their own behavior without much parental guidance or intervention

Down

2. Blood relationships
4. Family interaction

❖ CHAPTER 4
Growth and Development of Children

1. Categorizing growth and behavior into approximate age stages:
   A. helps to account for individual differences in children.
   B. can be applied to all children with some degree of precision.
   C. provides a convenient means to describe the majority of children.
   D. determines the speed of each child's growth.

2. Which of the following terms is correct to describe the period of rapid growth rate and total dependency that occurs between 8 weeks after conception until birth?
   A. prenatal
   B. germinal
   C. embryonic
   D. fetal

3. Which of the following is an example of a cephalocaudal directional trend in development?
   A. Infants stand after they are able to hold their back erect.
   B. Fingers and toes develop after embryonic limb buds.
   C. Infants manipulate fingers after they are able to use the whole hand as a unit.
   D. Infants begin to have fine muscle control after gross random muscle movement is established.

4. The directional trend that predicts an orderly and continuous development is known as:
   A. cephalocaudal.
   B. proximodistal.
   C. sequential.
   D. differentiation.

5. Which of the following is considered fixed and precise?
   A. the pace and rate of development
   B. the order of development
   C. physical growth, in particular, height
   D. growth during the vulnerable period

6. Sensitive periods in development are those times when the child is:
   A. more likely to respond to beneficial stimulation.
   B. more likely to require specific stimulation for physical growth.
   C. less likely to acquire a specific skill if it is not learned during this time.
   D. less likely to be harmed by external conditions.

7. Which of the following statements about individual differences in growth and development is FALSE?
   A. The pubescent growth spurt begins early in some children.
   B. Females reach their terminal height before males.
   C. Males reach their terminal height before females.
   D. Males reach their terminal weight after females.

8. Match the developmental trend in external proportions with the age group.

A. fetal

_____ Rapid growth and growth of the trunk with a high center of gravity predominates in this age group.

B. newborn

_____ The lower limbs constitute one half of the total body height and 30% of the total body weight.

C. infancy

_____ The head is the fastest growing part of the body; at one point during this stage the head constitutes 50% of the total body length.

D. childhood

_____ The legs are the most rapidly growing part of the body; and the slender, long-legged build is characteristic of both sexes during this stage.

E. adolescent

_____ The lower limbs are one third of the total body length but only 15% of the total body weight in this age group.

F. adult

_____ A large portion of the increase in height during this stage is the result of trunk elongation. The feet and hands also grow rapidly and may appear large and ungainly in proportion to the rest of the body.

9. Which of the following growth patterns is considerably greater in the male adolescent compared with the female adolescent?
   A. shoulder and hip growth
   B. anterior hip diameter
   C. the width of the pelvis
   D. the deposition of body fat

10. At birth, the infant brain has achieved what percent of its adult size?
   A. 90%
   B. 50%
   C. 25%
   D. 98%

11. The lordosis that a 15-month-old child develops would be considered a secondary curvature that is:
   A. located in the cervical region.
   B. fused and permanently fixed.
   C. a sign of a developmental delay.
   D. a compensatory lumbar curve exaggeration.

12. The maximum skeletal growth measure by linear growth or weight occurs:
   A. between ages 3 and 9 years.
   B. between ages 2 and 4 years.
   C. in the newborn stage.
   D. before birth.

13. If the height of a 2-year-old is measured as 88 cm, his height at adulthood may be estimated to be:
   A. 132 cm.
   B. 176 cm.
   C. 172 cm.
   D. 190 cm.

14. If a newborn measures 19 inches at birth, the expected height at age 4 years would be approximately:
    A. 28.5 inches.
    B. 38 inches.
    C. 43.5 inches.
    D. 48 inches.

15. At 17 years of age a girl will be considered to be at her:
    A. midgrowth height.
    B. terminal height.
    C. growth spurt.
    D. transitory height.

16. The 6-year molar is often used as a criterion for:
    A. developmental assessment.
    B. bone age.
    C. biologic age.
    D. certain endocrine problems.

17. The BEST estimate of biologic age can be made using measurements obtained from:
    A. nasal bone height.
    B. facial bone radiography.
    C. hand and wrist radiography.
    D. mandibular size.

18. Increasingly complex movement and neurologic changes in the infant can be attributed to the:
    A. rapid growth of the nervous system after birth.
    B. dramatic increase in the number of neurons immediately after birth.
    C. new nerve cells that appear after the sixth month of life.
    D. increasingly intricate communications with other cells.

19. The acquisition of motor skills depends primarily on the:
    A. myelinization and maturation of the nerve tracts.
    B. amount of stimulation the nerve tracts receive.
    C. influences of the environmental stimuli.
    D. persistence of primitive reflexes.

20. One probable reason for large lymph node development in the child is that lymph tissues growth patterns reflect the:
    A. parallel development of the nervous system.
    B. general growth patterns of the child.
    C. repeated exposure to new infectious agents.
    D. parallel development of the thymus gland.

21. When children experience a secondary cause of growth deficiency such as prematurity, they usually lag behind age mates in their developmental milestones until about the age of:
    A. 6 months.
    B. 2 years.
    C. 4 years.
    D. 6 years.

22. The daily requirement for dietary protein intake is lowest for which one of the following groups?
    A. adult males
    B. infants over 6 months of age
    C. school-age children
    D. infants under 6 months of age

23. The nurse determines that a 7-month-old infant who weighs 10 kg needs about:
    A. 450 kcal per day.
    B. 700 kcal per day.
    C. 1000 kcal per day.
    D. 1200 kcal per day.

24. The basal metabolic rate (BMR) is highest in the:
    A. adult male.
    B. infant over 6 months of age.
    C. school-age child.
    D. infant under 6 months of age.

25. The energy requirement to build tissue:
    A. fluctuates randomly.
    B. fluctuates based on need.
    C. steadily decreases with age.
    D. steadily increases with age.

26. Body temperature in young children and infants responds to:
    A. changes in the environment.
    B. exercise.
    C. emotional upset.
    D. all of the above.

27. Which one of the following motor behaviors is considered a general fundamental skill?
    A. jumping
    B. maturation of muscles
    C. rudimentary movement
    D. all of the above

28. The length of time spent in sleep increases somewhat:
    A. throughout childhood.
    B. during the pubertal growth spurt.
    C. by the age of 3 years.
    D. by the age of 18 months.

29. The rapid eye movement (REM) sleep of newborns consists of _____ percent of their sleep time.

30. A mother asks whether her child's sleep behavior is abnormal because he usually arouses during the night, looks around, and speaks unintelligibly. The nurse's response would be based on the knowledge that periodic wakening indicates that the child:
    A. has normal sleep behavior.
    B. has periods of sleeplessness.
    C. is slow to return to sleep.
    D. was very fatigued.

31. If parenting skills are lacking, the child's behavior may be perceived by the parent as:
    A. less difficult.
    B. easier.
    C. more distracted.
    D. more difficult.

32. Match the attribute of temperament with its description.

A. activity

    _____ amount of stimulation required to evoke a response

B. rhythmicity

    _____ nature of initial responses to a new stimulus: positive or negative

C. approach-withdrawal

    _____ regularity in the timing of physiologic functions such as hunger, sleep, and elimination

D. adaptability

    _____ energy level of the child's reactions

E. threshold of responsiveness

    _____ level of physical motion during activity

F. intensity of reaction

    _____ ease or difficulty with which the child adapts or adjusts to new situations

G. mood

H. distractibility

    _____ length of time a child pursues a given activity and continues

I. attention span and persistence

    _____ ease with which attention can be diverted

    _____ amount of pleasant behavior compared with the unpleasant

33. The term "difficult child" is a category derived by the individual's overall pattern of temperamental attributes that may:
    A. be used to categorize about 40% of all children.
    B. indicate that the child is even-tempered.
    C. indicate that the child has a poor "fit" with his/her environment.
    D. affect the child's adjustment throughout childhood.

34. Assessment of temperament provides useful information for anticipating probable areas of:
    A. maladaptive functioning.
    B. developmental risk.
    C. demand for adaptation.
    D. parental dissonance.

35. Personality development as viewed by Freud focuses on:
    A. the desire to satisfy biological needs.
    B. the suppression of psychosexual instincts.
    C. direct observations of adults.
    D. retrospective studies of children.

36. Erikson's theory provides a framework for:
    A. clearly indicating the experience needed to resolve crises.
    B. emphasizing pathologic development.
    C. coping with extraordinary events.
    D. explaining children's behavior in mastering developmental tasks.

37. Erikson's stage trust vs. mistrust corresponds to Freud's:
    A. anal stage.
    B. oral stage.
    C. phallic stage.
    D. guilt stage.

38. For adolescents, their struggle to fit the roles they have played and those they hope to play is best outlined by:
    A. Freud's latency period.
    B. Freud's phallic stage.
    C. Erikson's identity vs. role confusion.
    D. Erikson's intimacy vs. isolation.

39. Sullivan's theory of interpersonal development:
    A. recognizes the importance of the biologic maturation process.
    B. recognizes interpersonal relationships between children.
    C. recognizes the importance of social approval in developing self-concept.
    D. explains how children acquire feelings of security.

40. The best-known theory regarding cognitive development was developed by:
    A. Sullivan.
    B. Kohlberg.
    C. Erikson.
    D. Piaget.

41. A schema according to Piaget is a:
    A. skill of organizing new knowledge.
    B. cognitive developmental stage.
    C. mechanism to move from one stage to the next.
    D. pattern of action or thought.

42. An important prerequisite for all other mental activity is the child's awareness that an object exists even though it is no longer visible. According to Piaget, this awareness is called:
    A. object permanence.
    B. logical thinking.
    C. egocentricity.
    D. reversibility.

43. The predominant characteristic of Piaget's preoperational period is egocentricity, which according to Piaget means:
    A. concrete and tangible reasoning.
    B. selfishness and self-centeredness.
    C. inability to see another's perspective.
    D. ability to make deductions and generalize.

44. The stages of moral development which allow for prediction of behavior but not for individual differences are outlined in the moral development theory according to:
    A. Fowler.
    B. Holstein.
    C. Gilligan.
    D. Kohlberg.

45. The difference between religion and spirituality is that spirituality:
    A. requires an organized set of practices.
    B. affects the whole person: mind, body, and spirit.
    C. ensures the individual's desire to differentiate right from wrong.
    D. ensures rational moral decision making.

46. Children learn most of the syntax structures of their native language by the age of:
    A. 2 years.
    B. 3 years.
    C. 5 years.
    D. 7 years.

47. Most learning theorists believe that language is acquired:
    A. as children hear simplified versions of adult speech.
    B. through the maturation of the nervous system.
    C. through the assistance of an inborn language acquisition mechanism.
    D. as children hear and respond to the speech of their companions.

48. Match the concept with its description.

    A. classical conditioning where two events evoke the same response

    B. use of rewards to encourage specific behavior

    C. role modeling

    D. knowledge of oneself that influences relationships with others

    E. a component of self-concept that encompasses the individual's attitude toward his/her own body

    F. the affective component of self-concept

    G. the process by which children internalize the same sex parent's values and outlook

    _____ gender identity

    _____ operant conditioning

    _____ self-concept

    _____ Pavlovian conditioning

    _____ body image

    _____ self-esteem

    _____ Bandura's observational learning

49. The gender label is:
    A. achieved early and subtly through imitation.
    B. should not be assigned until at least 3 years of age.
    C. is affected primarily by the chromosomal determination of sex.
    D. only a small component of the child's total identity.

50. Match the type of play with the example of that type of play.

    A. sense pleasure   _____ coloring a picture

    B. skill play   _____ rocking a doll

    C. unoccupied behavior   _____ daydreaming

    D. dramatic play   _____ peekaboo/pattycake

    E. games   _____ watching *Sesame Street* on television

    F. onlooker play   _____ preparing a puppet show

    G. solitary play   _____ learning to ride a bicycle

    H. parallel play   _____ swinging

    I. associative play   _____ playing with dolls

    J. cooperative play   _____ toddlers playing blocks in the same room

51. Which of the following functions of play may be hindered by increasing the early academic achievements of a child?
    A. intellectual development
    B. creative development
    C. sensorimotor development
    D. moral development

52. Match the stage with the example of an appropriate toy for that stage.

    A. exploratory stage   _____   a deck of cards

    B. toy stage   _____   popular magazines to browse through

    C. play stage   _____   a tool box and tools

    D. daydreaming stage   _____   a busy box

53. The influence of heredity on behavior characteristics and intelligence is based on the:
    A. action of environment on heredity.
    B. action of heredity on environment.
    C. interaction between the environment and heredity.
    D. influence of environmental stimulation on achievement.

54. Which one of the following endocrine hormones has NOT been demonstrated to stimulate growth?
    A. glucagon
    B. growth hormone
    C. thyroid hormone
    D. androgen

55. Based on documented research, which one of the following behaviors can be attributed more to girls than to boys during childhood?
    A. more analytic
    B. lower self-esteem
    C. physical aggressiveness
    D. verbal aggressiveness

56. Based on documented research, which one of the following behaviors can be attributed more to boys than to girls?
    A. more analytic
    B. lower self-esteem
    C. physical aggressiveness
    D. verbal aggressiveness

57. Altered growth and development would be LEAST likely to be noteworthy in which one of the following disorders?
    A. chromosome abnormalities
    B. acute appendicitis
    C. chronic hepatitis
    D. cystic fibrosis

58. Match the growth or developmental influence with the example or description.

A. prenatal influences

B. altitude

C. environmental hazards

D. socioeconomic level

E. nutrition

F. love

G. significant others

H. security

I. discipline

J. independence

K. emotional deprivation

_____ protects children from dangers

_____ lead, pollution, radiation

_____ There are often great fluctuations in the development of this ability.

_____ the single most important emotional need for growth

_____ the single most important influence on growth

_____ play an important role in personality and intellectual development

_____ Hypoxia may limit development.

_____ occurs in homes with disorganized, distorted parent-child relationships

_____ General health and nutrition vary.

_____ Most childhood behavior problems are associated with the lack of this influencing factor.

_____ smoking/fetal alcohol

59. In relation to stress in childhood, it is MOST desirable to:
A. identify all of the possible childhood stressors.
B. provide children with interpersonal security.
C. protect children from stressors.
D. realize that most children are not vulnerable to stress.

60. Which one of the following coping strategies would be considered an example of primary control?
A. listening to music
B. submission
C. withdrawal
D. tantrums

61. The medium that has the MOST impact on children in America today is:
A. television.
B. movies.
C. comic books.
D. newspapers.

❖ Critical Thinking ❖
Case Study

Brian Adams, who is 8 years old, arrives at the clinic for a checkup for school. He has historically been in the 50th percentile for both height and weight and is generally considered healthy. He has a family history of heart disease.

Mrs. Adams is concerned about an increase in her son's physical aggressiveness lately. Today Brian's height is noted to be in the 50th percentile, but his weight is in the 95th percentile. His mother states that he watches television each day. His serum cholesterol level is elevated.

62. Based on the information in the case study above, the nurse would estimate that:
    A. Brian is exposed to only the positive effects of television.
    B. using family history of heart disease is an excellent screening indicator for cholesterol testing.
    C. Brian probably watches more than two hours of television per day.
    D. there is no link between Brian's television viewing and his increased physical aggression.

63. Based on the assessment information presented about Brian, which one of the following nursing diagnoses would be MOST appropriate?
    A. altered growth and development
    B. altered nutrition: less than body requirements
    C. fluid volume excess
    D. altered parenting

64. Which one of the following interventions in regard to Brian's television viewing would be LEAST appropriate for the nurse to suggest?
    A. Restrict Brian's viewing of violent programs.
    B. Watch Brian's favorite shows with him each day.
    C. Help Brian to correlate consequences with actions and point out subtle messages.
    D. Explore alternatives to aggressive conflict resolution.

65. Which of the following outcomes would be BEST to expect in regard to Brian?
    A. Brian's aggressive behavior decreases significantly, his intake of high-cholesterol snacks decreases, and his television viewing time decreases.
    B. Brian is able to explain the television programs that he watches.
    C. Brian selects more healthful snacks and watches television about one hour per day.
    D. Brian's cholesterol decreases to normal level, his weight is at the 50th percentile, and his mother reports that his aggressive behavior is decreased.

❖ *Crossword Puzzle* ❖

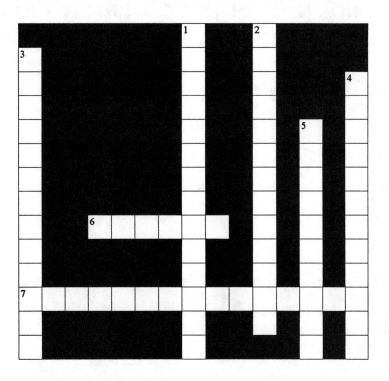

Across

6. An increase in number and size of cells
7. Processes by which early cells and structures are systematically modified and altered to achieve specific and characteristic properties

Down

1. Method of child study that measures a group of children at the same point in time
2. Near-to-far direction of growth
3. Head-to-tail direction of growth
4. A method of child study that compares the same child at different points in time
5. An increase in competence and adaptability; aging

❖ CHAPTER 5
Hereditary Influences on Health Promotion of the Child and Family

1. Trisomy 21 or Down syndrome is an example of a(n):
   A. congenital chromosomal association.
   B. sex chromosome abnormality.
   C. autoimmune aberration.
   D. autosomal structural aberration.

2. All of the following chromosomal disorders are considered sex chromosome abnormalities EXCEPT:
   A. Turner syndrome.
   B. Klinefelter syndrome.
   C. cri du chat syndrome.
   D. triple X syndrome.

3. The Lyon hypothesis helps to explain why children with sex chromosome abnormalities compared with children with autosomal abnormalities:
   A. usually have milder physical and mental deficiencies.
   B. are shorter in stature with poor coordination.
   C. are more easily identified at birth.
   D. usually have more severe handicaps.

4. Which one of the following types of congenital defects is more characteristically caused by recessive genes?
   A. structural
   B. metabolic

5. Match the disorder with the inheritance pattern. (Inheritance patterns may be used more than once.)

   A. autosomal dominant   _____ Wilson disease

   B. autosomal recessive   _____ Tay-Sachs disease

   C. sex-linked (dominant or recessive) _____ osteogenesis imperfecta

                                   _____ neurofibromatosis

                                   _____ Duchenne muscular dystrophy

                                   _____ maple syrup urine disease

                                   _____ hemophilia A

                                   _____ fragile X syndrome

                                   _____ ocular albinism

                                   _____ achondroplasia

                                   _____ cystic fibrosis

_____ galactosemia

_____ familial hypothyroidism

_____ Marfan syndrome

_____ myotonic dystrophy

_____ Noonan syndrome

_____ phenylketonuria

_____ thalassemias

6. A disease or defect that is encountered frequently in the population without a clear-cut inheritance pattern would be classified as:
   A. mutation.
   B. mosaicism.
   C. uniparental disomy.
   D. multifactorial.

7. Which one of the following disorders has no clear relationship to the HLA (human leukocyte antigen)?
   A. type I diabetes
   B. rheumatoid arthritis
   C. fetal alcohol syndrome
   D. myasthenia gravis

8. Fetal surgery has been used in particular to treat congenital:
   A. urinary tract abnormalities.
   B. heart disease.
   C. facial and limb deformities.
   D. pyloric stenosis.

9. Phenylketonuria is usually treated by:
   A. diet modification.
   B. hormone replacement.
   C. surgical repair.
   D. vitamin supplement.

10. Careful counseling is necessary when screening an individual for carrier status of hereditary disorders because:
    A. this type of screening is controversial.
    B. of possible ethical dilemmas.
    C. this type of screening is expensive.
    D. the emotional threat for the child is always devastating.

11. Which one of the following statements is NOT a part of the controversial aspect of mass genetic screening programs?
    A. Health professionals sometimes lack knowledge about the purpose of the testing.
    B. The public cost of testing does not always outweigh the benefits.
    C. Many well-organized programs have been successful in preventing disease.
    D. The psychological implications of the carrier states can be handled improperly.

12. Match the type of prenatal genetic test with its purpose.

A. maternal serum alpha-fetoprotein (MS-AFP) _____   to perform chromosome and biochemical analysis

B. ultrasonography _____   to estimate gestational age and identify structural abnormalities

C. amniocentesis

_____   to perform chromosomal analysis at the earliest possible point during pregnancy

D. chorionic villus sampling (CVS)

_____   to screen for neural tube defects

13. Preimplantation genetic diagnosis has been used for parents at risk of having a child with:
    A. Down syndrome.
    B. a neural tube defect.
    C. a congenital heart defect.
    D. cystic fibrosis.

14. Which of the following actions would NOT be considered an appropriate nursing responsibility in genetic counseling?
    A. Choose the best course of action for the family.
    B. Identify families who would benefit from genetic evaluation.
    C. Become familiar with community resources for genetic evaluation.
    D. Learn basic genetic principles.

15. The most efficient genetic counseling service provided by a group of genetic screening specialists may:
    A. predict the outcome of the disease.
    B. take less than two hours.
    C. evaluate the affected child only.
    D. be inaccessible to the people who need it most.

16. *Proband* is the term used in genetic counseling that means the:
    A. affected person.
    B. genetic history.
    C. clinical manifestations.
    D. mode of inheritance.

17. When teaching families about genetic risks and probabilities, the nurse may need to:
    A. make specific recommendations.
    B. use games such as flipping coins and horse racing.
    C. realize that most people have a basic understanding of biology.
    D. recognize that each pregnancy's probabilities build on the previous pregnancy's probabilities.

18. Which one of the following assessment findings would alert the nurse to the need for genetic counseling?
    A. individuals with a family history of tuberculosis
    B. parents who had an infant born at 42 weeks' gestation
    C. couples with a history of infertility
    D. pregnant adolescents

19. Which one of the following assessment findings in an infant would indicate to the nurse that there is a need for genetic referral?
    A. vernix caseosa
    B. acrocyanosis
    C. mongolian spots
    D. odorous breath

20. When drawing a pedigree genogram, which one of the following facts would be LEAST significant? The proband's:
    A. paternal grandmother had two stillbirth pregnancies.
    B. sibling died as an infant in a motor vehicle accident.
    C. paternal grandfather was a carrier for sickle cell disease.
    D. half-brother carries the sickle cell trait.

21. Which one of the following statements in regard to genetic counseling is FALSE?
    A. Families have a tendency to be more ashamed of a hereditary disorder than other illness.
    B. The nurse's role in genetic counseling involves sympathy and supportive listening.
    C. The nurse ensures that clients have accurate and complete information to make decisions.
    D. Most couples will choose not to have a child if there is any risk of disability.

❖ Critical Thinking ❖
Case Study

Mr. and Mrs. Jones are waiting in the obstetrician's office for a routine prenatal checkup. The couple is Roman Catholic and do not believe in abortion. The obstetrician has recommended a screening test to rule out neural tube defects. Mrs. Jones does not see any benefit from this testing procedure and does not want to undergo the procedure.

22. Which one of the following factors is the LEAST important consideration during the assessment phase of this visit?
    A. The nurse is not Roman Catholic.
    B. The test is a venipuncture and carries little risk.
    C. Most couples receive normal results from prenatal tests.
    D. Results of the tests will be provided before the delivery date.

23. Which one of the following considerations should the nurse deal with first?
    A. The couple believes that testing is used to identify anomalies in order to terminate pregnancies.
    B. The couple's clear-cut beliefs about pregnancy termination are very different from the reality of raising an abnormal child.
    C. The nurse believes that pregnancy termination for fetal abnormalities is often the best option.
    D. The nurse believes that raising a child with a terminal illness is extremely difficult.

24. Which one of the following goals would be MOST appropriate for the nurse in this situation?
    A. to provide nonjudgmental supportive counseling
    B. to help the couple make their decision
    C. to provide follow-up care to the couple
    D. to educate the couple about neural tube defects

25. Which of the following statements by Mrs. Jones indicates that the nurse's goal was met?
    A. "I had no idea what was involved in raising a disabled child."
    B. "Your ideas have been very helpful. I think one of them will work."
    C. "We will discuss this and call you tomorrow with our decision."
    D. "I had no idea what neural tube defects were."

❖ *Crossword Puzzle* ❖

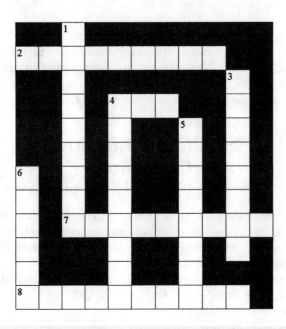

Across

2. A condition or trait produced by environmental factors that cannot be distinguished from one due to genetic factors
4. Phenylketonuria
7. The science concerned with improvement of the human race through control of environmental factors
8. A condition present at birth

Down

1. Refers to a gene that is expressed only when it is present in the homozygous state
3. The science concerned with improving the genetic potential of the human population by control of heredity through voluntary social action
4. The physical or chemical characteristics of an individual
5. Refers to a gene that produces an effect (is expressed) whenever it is present
6. Presence of two or more genotypically different cell lines in the same individual

❖ CHAPTER 6
Communication and Health Assessment of the Child and Family

1. Which nursing action would negatively affect the communication process between the nurse and the client?
   A. Messages delivered to the client are congruous.
   B. Communication includes the child as well as the parent.
   C. The nurse uses verbal and nonverbal communication to reflect approval of the client's statement.
   D. The nurse uses a slow, even, steady voice to convey instruction.

2. Mrs. Green has brought her daughter Karen to the clinic as a new patient. Karen, age 12 years, requires a physical examination so that she can play volleyball. Which one of the following techniques used by the nurse to establish effective communication during the interview process is NOT correct?
   A. The nurse introduces himself/herself and asks the name of all family members present.
   B. After the introduction, the nurse is careful to direct questions about Karen to Mrs. Green since she is the best source of information.
   C. After the introduction and explanation of her role, the nurse begins the interview by saying to Karen, "Tell me about your volleyball team."
   D. The nurse chooses to conduct the interview in a quiet area with few distractions.

3. While conducting an assessment of the child, the nurse communicates with the child's family. Which one of the following does the nurse recognize as NOT productive in obtaining information?
   A. obtaining input from the child, verbal and nonverbal
   B. observing the relationship between parents and child
   C. using broad, open-ended questions
   D. avoiding the use of guiding statements to direct the focus of the interview

4. The capacity to understand what another person is feeling by experiencing from that person's frame of reference is described as:
   A. sympathy.
   B. empathy.
   C. reassurance.
   D. encouragement.

5. Anticipatory guidance should:
   A. view family weakness as a competence builder.
   B. focus on problem resolution.
   C. base interventions on needs identified by the nurse.
   D. empower the family to use information to build parenting ability.

6. The nurse recognizes which of the following statements as TRUE and which as FALSE when planning how to communicate effectively with children?

   _____ Nonverbal components of the communication process do not convey significant messages.

   _____ Children are alert to their surroundings and attach meaning to gestures.

   _____ Active attempts to make friends with children before they have had an opportunity to evaluate an unfamiliar person increases their anxiety.

   _____ The nurse should assume a position that is at eye level with the child.

_____ Communication through transition objects such as dolls or stuffed animals delays the child's response to verbal communication offered by the nurse.

7. Communication with children must reflect their developmental thought process. Match the development stage with the description of communication guidelines to be used. (Stages may be used more than once.)

A. infancy

B. early childhood

C. school-age years

D. adolescence

_____ focus communication on the child; experiences of others are of no interest to them

_____ primarily use and respond to nonverbal communication

_____ interpret words literally and are unable to separate fact from fantasy

_____ assign human attributes to inanimate objects

_____ require explanations and reasons why procedures are being done to them

_____ have a heightened concern about body integrity, being overly sensitive to any activity that constitutes a threat to it

_____ often willing to discuss their concern with an adult outside the family and often welcome the opportunity to interact with a nurse

8. Which one of the following BEST describes the appropriate use of play as a communication technique in children?
   A. Small infants have little response to activities that focus on repetitive actions like patting and stroking.
   B. Few clues about intellectual or social developmental progress are obtained from the observation of a child's play behaviors.
   C. Therapeutic play has little value in reduction of trauma from illness or hospitalization.
   D. Play sessions serve as assessment tools for determining children's awareness and perception of illness.

9. Several creative communication techniques are often used with children. Identify which is being used in each of the following examples.

   _____ A. The nurse shows Tina a picture of a child having an intravenous infusion started and asks Tina to describe the scene.

   _____ B. "I am concerned about how the medicine treatments are going because I want you to feel better."

   _____ C. The nurse reads Tina a story from a book and asks her to retell the story.

   _____ D. The nurse provides Tina with crayons and paper and asks her to draw a picture of her family.

   _____ E. The nurse gives Tina a doll and a stethoscope and allows Tina to listen to the doll's heart.

10. A complete pediatric health history includes ten expected components. List these components.

   _____   _____

   _____   _____

   _____   _____

   _____   _____

11. In eliciting the chief complaint, the nurse identifies which one of the following techniques as NOT appropriate?
    A. limiting the chief complaint to a brief statement restricted to one or two symptoms
    B. using labeling-type questions such as "How are you sick?" to facilitate information exchange
    C. recording the chief complaint in the child's or parent's own words
    D. using open-ended neutral questions to elicit information

12. Which component of the pediatric health history is the following? "Nausea and vomiting for three days. Started with abdominal cramping past eating hamburger at home. No pain or cramping at present. Unable to keep any foods down but able to drink clear liquids without vomiting. No temperature elevation, no diarrhea."
    A. chief complaint
    B. past history
    C. present illness
    D. review of systems

13. The nurse recognizes which one of the following as NOT part of the past history included in a pediatric health history?
    A. symptom analysis
    B. allergies
    C. birth history
    D. current medications

14. The nurse knows that the BEST description of the sexual history for a pediatric health history:
    A. includes a discussion of plans for future children.
    B. allows the client to introduce sexual activity history.
    C. includes a discussion of contraception methods only when the client discloses current sexual activity.
    D. alerts the nurse to the need for sexually transmitted disease screening.

15. The _____ uses symbols to diagram data about the family structure.

    The _____ records the family medical history in chart form.

    The _____ is a visual presentation of the family's support system.

16. Indications for the nurse to conduct a comprehensive family assessment include which of the following?
    1. children with developmental delays
    2. children with history of repeated accidental injuries
    3. children with behavioral problems
    4. children receiving comprehensive well-child care
    A. 1, 2, 3, and 4
    B. 2, 3, and 4
    C. 1 and 2
    D. 2 and 3

17. Assessment of family structure is BEST conducted:
    A. after the first meeting with the client.
    B. only when a problem is suspected within the family.
    C. towards the end of the interview when rapport has been established.
    D. by interviewing the client about other family members' roles within the family.

18. Assessment of family interactions and roles, decision making and problem solving, and communication is known as assessment of:
    A. family structure.
    B. family function.
    C. family composition.
    D. home and community environment.

19. The dietary history of a pediatric client includes:
    A. a 12-hour dietary intake recall.
    B. a more specific, detailed history for the older child.
    C. financial and cultural factors that influence food selection.
    D. criticism of parents' allowance of non-essential foods.

❖ Critical Thinking ❖
Case Study

Mrs. Brown brings her 11-year-old son, Kenny, to the clinic for a physical. She is concerned because Kenny comes home from school "very tired and only wants to watch television." Kenny's bedtime has not changed, he performs well in school, and his mother denies stress or problems within the home. On physical examination, Kenny is above the 90th percentile for weight by 25 pounds.

20. To effectively establish a setting for communication, the nurse, upon entering the room with Mrs. Brown and Kenny, introduces herself and explains her role and the purpose of the interview. Kenny is included in the interaction as the nurse asks his name and age and what he is expecting at his visit today. The nurse next informs Mrs. Brown and Kenny that Kenny is 25 pounds overweight and that his diet and exercise plan must be "terrible" for Kenny to be in "such bad shape." Which aspect of effective communication has the nurse forgotten that will MOST significantly impact the exchange of information during this interview?
    A. assurance of privacy and confidentiality
    B. preliminary acquaintance
    C. directing the focus away from the complaint of fatigue to one of obesity
    D. injecting her own attitudes and feelings into the interview

21. Based on the information provided, the nurse can correctly record which of the following?
    A. chief complaint
    B. present illness
    C. past medical history
    D. symptom analysis

22. Mrs. Brown, Kenny, and the nurse agree to the need to conduct a more intensive nutritional assessment. Which one of the following ways to record Kenny's dietary intake would the nurse suggest as MOST reliable in providing needed information to currently assess Kenny's dietary habits?
    A 12-hour recall
    B. 24-hour recall
    C. food diary for 3-day period
    D. food frequency questionnaire

23. The nurse explains to Mrs. Brown and to Kenny that part of the nutritional status examination will include measure-

    ments of skinfold thickness and arm circumference. These are done to _____

    _____ _____ _____ and are part of the clinical examination

    known as _____.

24. The physical examination has been completed to reflect that other than his obesity, Kenny is in excellent physical health with normal blood counts. The completed nutritional assessment reflects that Mrs. Brown and Kenny have little knowledge about proper nutrition and that Kenny has a large intake of "junk" foods high in fat and calories but low in nutrients. Based on the data collected, which one of the following nursing diagnoses would be MOST appropriate?
    A. altered family processes related to parents' knowledge deficit
    B. altered family coping related to family's inability to purchase needed foods
    C. altered individual coping related to fatigue from poor dietary habits
    D. altered nutrition: more than body requirements related to eating practices

❖ Crossword Puzzle ❖

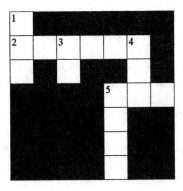

Across

2. Family Adaptability, Partnership, Growth, Affection, and Resolve
5. Home screening questionnaire

Down

1. Kinetic family drawing
3. Present illness
4. Review of systems
5. Home Observation and Measurement of the Environment

❖ CHAPTER 7
Physical and Developmental Assessment of the Child

1. In examining pediatric clients, the normal sequence of head-to-toe direction is often altered to accommodate the client's developmental needs. The nurse identifies which of the following goals as LEAST likely to guide the examination process?
   A. Minimize the stress and anxiety associated with the assessment of body parts.
   B. Record the findings according to the normal sequence.
   C. Foster a trusting nurse-child relationship.
   D. Preserve the essential security of the parent-child relationship.

2. Mr. Alls brings his son, Keith, in for Keith's regular well infant examination. Keith is 12 months old. The nurse knows that the BEST approach to the physical examination for this client will be to:
   A. have the infant sit in the parent's lap to complete as much of the examination as possible.
   B. place the infant on the examining table with parent out of view.
   C. perform examination in head-to-toe direction.
   D. completely undress Keith and leave him undressed during the examination.

3. Behavior that signals the child's readiness to cooperate during the physical examination would NOT include:
   A. talking to the nurse.
   B. making eye contact with the nurse.
   C. allowing physical touching.
   D. sitting on parent's lap, playing with doll.

4. The National Center for Health Statistics has growth charts available for pediatric clients. A major difference between

   the age-related charts is that the chart for ages birth to 36 months records height as _____

   _____ while the chart for ages 2 to 18 years records height as _____ .

5. The assessment method that the nurse expects to provide the BEST information about the physical growth pattern of a preschool-age child is:
   A. recording height and weight measurements of the child on the standardized percentile growth chart.
   B. keeping a flow sheet for height, weight, and head circumference increases.
   C. obtaining a history of sibling growth patterns.
   D. measuring the height, weight, and head circumference of the child.

6. Identify the following statements regarding the growth or development patterns of pediatric clients as either TRUE or FALSE.

   _____ Comparing children's growth trends with those of their parents is essential in evaluating adequate growth.

   _____ Breast-fed infants grow faster than bottle-fed infants during the 6- to 18-month age period.

   _____ Growth is a continuous but uneven process, and the most reliable evaluation lies in comparison of growth measurements over a prolonged time.

   _____ Growth measurements during the physical examination should be age-specific and include length, height, weight, skinfold thickness, and arm and head circumference.

7. Head circumference is:
   A. measured in all children up to the age of 24 months.
   B. equal to chest circumference at about 1 to 2 years of age.
   C. about 8 to 9 cm smaller than chest circumference during childhood.
   D. measured slightly below the eyebrows and pinna of the ears.

8. In infants and small children, the _____ pulse should be taken because it is the most reliable. This

   pulse should be counted for _____ _____ _____ because of the possibility of
   irregularities in rhythm.

9. Which one of the following findings would the nurse recognize as normal when measuring the vital signs of a 9-year-old child?
   A. femoral pulses graded at +1
   B. oral temperature of 100.9° F
   C. blood pressure of 101/61
   D. respiratory rate of 28

10. The nurse knows to eliminate which of the following observations when recording the general appearance of the child?
    A. impression of child's nutritional status
    B. behavior, interactions with parents
    C. hygiene, cleanliness
    D. vital signs

11. Match the skin assessment finding or description with the terminology. (A term may be used more than once.)

    A. cyanosis   _____   appears in dark-skinned clients as ashen-gray lips and tongue

    B. pallor   _____   appears in light-skinned clients as purplish to yellow-green areas

    C. erythema   _____   may be a sign of anemia, chronic disease, edema, or shock

    D. ecchymosis   _____   redness of the skin which may be the result of infection, local inflammation,
                                    or increased temperature from climatic conditions
    E. petechiae
                           _____   large, diffuse areas, usually blue or black in color and the result of injury
    F. jaundice
                           _____   small, distinct pinpoint hemorrhages

                           _____   yellow staining of the skin usually caused by bile pigments

12. The nurse is assessing skin turgor in 10-month-old Ryan. The nurse grasps the skin on the abdomen between the thumb and index finger, pulls it taut, and quickly releases it. The tissue remains suspended or tented for a few seconds, then slowly falls back on the abdomen. Which of the following evaluations can the nurse correctly assume?
    A. The tissue shows normal elasticity.
    B. The child is properly hydrated.
    C. The assessment was done incorrectly.
    D. The child has poor skin turgor.

13. The nurse is assessing 7-year-old Mary's lymph nodes. The nurse uses the distal portions of his fingers and gently but firmly presses in a circular motion along the occipital and postauricular node areas. The nurse records the findings as "tender, enlarged warm lymph nodes." The nurse knows that the:
    A. findings are within normal limits for Mary's age.
    B. assessment technique was incorrect and should be repeated.
    C. findings suggest infection or inflammation in the scalp area or external ear canal.
    D. recording of the information is complete because it includes temperature and tenderness.

14. The nurse recognizes that an assessment finding of the head and neck which does NOT need referral is:
    A. head lag before 6 months of age.
    B. hyperextension of the head with pain on flexion.
    C. palpable thyroid gland including isthmus and lobes.
    D. closure of the anterior fontanel at the age of 9 months.

15. Sinuses that are present soon after birth are the _____ and _____ sinuses.

16. Normal findings on examination of the pupil may be recorded as PERRLA, which means

    _____.

17. Which one of the following assessments is an expected finding in the child's eye examination?
    A. opaque red reflex of the eye
    B. ophthalmoscopic examination reflects veins are darker in color and about one fourth larger in size than the arteries
    C. strabismus in the 12-month-old infant
    D. 5-year-old child who reads the Snellen eye chart at the 20/40 level

18. When assessing the ear in the 2-year-old child, the nurse should:
    A. expect cerumen in the external ear canal.
    B. use the smallest speculum to prevent trauma to the ear.
    C. pull the pinna up and back to better visualize the canal.
    D. pull the pinna down and back to better visualize the canal.

19. The test that measures the compliance of the tympanic membrane and the middle ear pressure is:
    A. Rinne test.
    B. threshold acuity sweep test.
    C. vestibular testing.
    D. tympanometry.

20. Four-year-old Billy has been brought to the clinic by his parents because they have noticed a sudden foul odor in the mouth accompanied by a discharge from the right nares. The nurse knows that this is MOST likely to suggest:
    A. poor dental hygiene.
    B. foreign body in the nose.
    C. gingival disease.
    D. thumb-sucking.

21. When assessing 4-year-old Gail's chest, the nurse would expect:
    A. movement of the chest wall to be symmetric bilaterally and coordinated with breathing.
    B. respiratory movements to be chiefly thoracic.
    C. anteroposterior diameter to be equal to the transverse diameter.
    D. retraction of the muscles between the ribs on respiratory movement.

22. The nurse asks 12-year-old Susan to repeat the word "99" several times while the palmar surfaces of the nurse's hands are placed on the child's chest. The nurse is palpating for conduction of sound through the respiratory tract. What is this called?
    A. pleural friction rub
    B. crepitation
    C. normal respiratory movements
    D. vocal fremitus

23. On auscultation of 8-year-old Tammie's lung fields, the nurse hears inspiratory sounds that are louder, longer, and higher-pitched than on expiration. These sounds are heard over the chest except over the scapula and sternum. These sounds are:
    A. bronchovesicular breath sounds.
    B. vesicular breath sounds.
    C. bronchial breath sounds.
    D. adventitious breath sounds.

24. When the nurse is palpating for cardiac thrills, the nurse knows that thrills are:
    A. vibrations caused by the flow of blood from one chamber to another through a narrowed opening.
    B. best felt with the dorsal surface of the hands.
    C. found at the point of maximum intensity.
    D. louder on inspiration than on expiration.

25. A heart sound that is the result of vibrations produced during ventricular filling and normally heard in some children is:
    A. S1.
    B. S2.
    C. S3.
    D. S4.

26. Examination of the abdomen is performed correctly by the nurse in the following order:
    A. inspection, palpation, percussion, and auscultation.
    B. inspection, percussion, auscultation, and palpation.
    C. palpation, percussion, auscultation, and inspection.
    D. inspection, auscultation, percussion, and palpation.

27. In performing an examination for scoliosis, the nurse understands that which one of the following is an INCORRECT method?
    A. The child should be examined only in his/her underpants (and bra if an older girl).
    B. The child should stand erect with the nurse observing from behind.
    C. The child should squat down with hands extended forward so that the nurse can observe for asymmetry of the shoulder blades.
    D. The child should bend forward so that the back is parallel to the floor and the nurse can observe from the side.

28. The Denver Developmental Screening Test is limited by its inability to predict:
    A. developmental delays in children of cultural ethnic groups.
    B. gross motor delays.
    C. language delays.
    D. personal-social delays.

❖ *Critical Thinking* ❖
Case Study

Mary, a 13-year-old, has come to the clinic with her mother with a complaint of right side abdominal pain of 24 hours' duration. She tells you, the nurse, that she has had some nausea and vomiting but no diarrhea. Her appetite is depressed and she feels hot and feverish. Mary has taken Tylenol for pain but with little relief.

29. In preparing Mary for physical examination, you know that during the examination, as an adolescent Mary will likely:
    A. prefer her parents to be present during the entire examination.
    B. desire to undress in private and will feel more comfortable when provided with a gown.
    C. prefer traumatic procedures such as ears and mouth examinations last.
    D. need to have heart and lungs auscultated first.

30. The nurse completes the physical examination and evaluates which of the following as an abnormal finding?
    A. Bowel sounds are stimulated by stroking the abdominal surface with the fingernail.
    B. Mary has no abdominal discomfort when she is supine with the legs flexed at the hips and knees.
    C. Mary's eyes are open during palpation of the abdomen.
    D. When the nurse presses firmly over the area distal to the right side of the abdomen and quickly releases this pressure, pain is intensified in the lower right side.

31. Which one of the following organs is located in the lower right quadrant of the abdomen?
    A. bladder
    B. liver
    C. ovaries
    D. appendix

32. Mary's parents are apprehensive about Mary and ask the nurse whether "it is serious." Which one of the following is the BEST response?
    A. "Mary has appendicitis and will need to have surgery immediately."
    B. "You will have to ask the doctor about her condition."
    C. "Mary has some abdominal pain which is not normal. We are watching her very carefully and will be able to tell you more when the laboratory tests are completed."
    D. "Mary should be able to go home as soon as the doctor finishes examining her and the laboratory tests are completed."

❖ Crossword Puzzle ❖

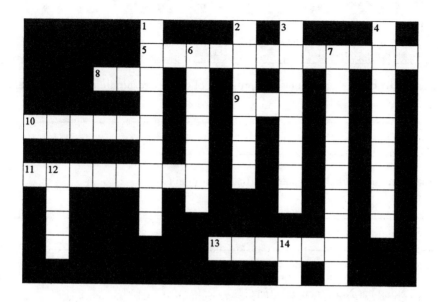

Across

5. Listening for sounds produced by the body
8. Midclavicular line
9. Intercostal space
10. Pupils equal, round, react to light and accommodation
11. Near the front of the body
13. Back of the eyeball

Down

1. Use of touch to detect structures of the skin
2. The external ear
3. Instrument used to view the interior of the ear
4. Nearer the back of the body
6. Standing height
7. Crosswise
12. National Center for Health Statistics
14. Disc diameter

❖ CHAPTER 8
Health Promotion of the Newborn and Family

1. The chemical factors in the blood that stimulate the initiation of the first respiration in the neonate are

   _____ _____, _____ _____

   _____, and _____ _____.

2. The primary thermal stimulus that helps initiate the first respiration is

   _____

   _____.

3. The nurse recognizes that tactile stimulation probably has some effect on initiation of respiration in the neonate. Which one of the following has NO beneficial effect?
   A. normal handling of the neonate
   B. drying the skin of the neonate
   C. slapping the neonate's heel or buttocks
   D. placing the infant skin to skin with the mother

4. The nurse knows which one of these neonates will MOST likely need additional respiratory support at birth?
   A. the infant born by normal vaginal delivery
   B. the infant born by cesarean birth
   C. the infant born vaginally after 12 hours of labor
   D. the infant born with high levels of surfactant

5. During the transition from fetal to neonatal circulation, the newborn's cardiovascular system accomplishes which of the following anatomic and physiologic alterations?
   1. closure of the ductus venosus
   2. closure of the foramen ovale
   3. closure of the ductus arteriosis
   4. increased systemic pressure and decreased pulmonary artery pressure
   A. 1, 2, 3, and 4
   B. 1, 2, and 3
   C. 2, 3, and 4
   D. 1, 3, and 4

6. Identify the following statements about infant adjustments to extrauterine life as either TRUE or FALSE.

   _____ Factors that predispose the neonate to excessive heat loss are large surface area, thin layer of subcutaneous fat, and the lack of shivering to produce heat.

   _____ Nonshivering thermogenesis is an effective method of heat production in the neonate since it is able to produce heat with little use of oxygen.

   _____ Brown fat or brown adipose tissue has a greater capacity to produce heat than does ordinary adipose tissue.

_____ The longer the infant is attached to the placenta, the less blood volume will be received by the neonate.

_____ Deficient production of pancreatic amylase impairs utilization of complex carbohydrates.

_____ Deficiency of pancreatic lipase assists the neonate in the digestion of cow's milk.

_____ Most salivary glands are functioning at birth even though most infants do not start drooling until teeth erupt.

_____ The stomach capacity for most newborn infants is about 90 cc.

_____ The newborn should be expected to void within the first 48 hours.

7. Match the term with its description.

A. meconium   _____ pale yellow to golden; pasty consistency

B. breast-fed infant stools   _____ first stool dark green; pasty, sticky consistency

C. formula-fed infant stools   _____ pale yellow to light brown; firmer in consistency with more offensive odor

8. Newborns receive passive immunity in the form of IgG from the _____ _____

and from _____ _____.

9. The nurse recognizes that all of the following effects of maternal sex hormones in the newborn are normal EXCEPT:
A. miniature puberty.
B. secretion of witch's milk from the newborn breasts.
C. pseudomenstruation.
D. bleeding from the breast nipples.

10. Fill in the blanks in the following statements as they pertain to sensory functions in the normal newborn.

A. The newborn can fixate on a bright object that is within _____ _____ and in the midline of the visual field.

B. Infants have visual preferences for the colors of _____, _____, and

_____ and for designs such as _____ _____ _____

_____.

C. The newborn's response to _____ frequency sounds is one of decreased motor activity and

crying while exposure to _____ frequency sound elicits an alerting reaction.

11. The nurse is performing the 5-minute Apgar on a newborn. Which one of the following observations is included in the Apgar score?
A. blood pressure
B. temperature
C. muscle tone
D. weight

12. Match the period of reactivity with the observations the nurse is likely to have during each period.

    A. first period of reactivity   _____   excellent bonding period and time to start breast-feeding

    B. second stage of first period of reactivity   _____   period of infant sleep lasting two to four hours; heart rate and respiratory rate decrease

    C. second period of reactivity

                                         _____   gastric and respiratory secretions are increased; passage of meconium commonly occurs

13. The nurse uses the Brazelton Neonatal Behavioral Assessment Scale to assess the newborn's behavioral responses. How would the nurse define *habituation*?
    A. responsiveness of the newborn to auditory and visual stimuli
    B. process whereby the newborn becomes accustomed to stimuli
    C. The infant is easily aroused from sleep state.
    D. The infant has a reactive Moro reflex with good muscle tone and coordination.

14. The nurse recognizes that one of the following is not correct about the relationship of newborn weight to gestational age. Which is FALSE?
    A. All infants under the weight of 2500 g (5 1/2 pounds) are premature by gestational age.
    B. Gestational age is more closely related to fetal maturity than is birth weight.
    C. Classification of infants by both weight and gestational age can be beneficial for predicting mortality risks.
    D. Heredity influences are a normal part of assessment.

15. On assessment of a 24-hour newborn, the nurse makes several observations. Which is normal?
    A. head circumference of 37 cm
    B. axillary temperature of 96° F
    C. Infant's posture is one of flexion of head and extremities, which rest on chest and abdomen.
    D. respirations of 68

16. Newborns lose up to 10% of their birth weight by 3 to 4 days of age. One factor that does NOT contribute to this process is:
    A. limited fluid intake in breast-fed infants.
    B. incomplete digestion of complex carbohydrates.
    C. loss of excessive extracellular fluid.
    D. passage of meconium.

17. When assessing blood pressure in the newborn, the nurse knows that which of the following is TRUE?
    A. A difference in systolic BP between the calf and upper arm in which the BP in the calf is 10 mm Hg less than in the upper arm needs referral.
    B. Routine BP measurements of full-term neonates are an excellent predictor of hypertension.
    C. A normal BP reading for a 3-day-old infant would be approximately 90/60.
    D. BP should be measured routinely on all healthy newborns as recommended by the American Academy of Pediatrics.

18. A widened, tense, bulging fontanel can be a sign of _____ _____

    _____ while a markedly sunken, depressed fontanel is a sign of _____.

19. Components of the physical assessment of the newborn include which of the following?
    1. clinical gestational age assessment
    2. general measurements
    3. general appearance
    4. head-to-toe assessment
    5. parent-infant attachment
    A. 1, 2, 3, 4, and 5
    B. 1, 2, 3, and 4
    C. 2, 3, 4, and 5
    D. 2, 3, and 4

20. Which of the following observations from the eye assessment of a newborn is recognized as normal?
    A. purulent discharge at age 48 hours
    B. absence of the red reflex at age 24 hours
    C. no pupillary reflex at age 3 weeks
    D. presence of strabismus at age 48 hours

21. It is important to assess for nasal patency in the newborn because newborns are

    _____.

22. The nurse correctly identifies the need to notify the physician for which neonate?
    A. the 24-hour-old neonate found to have Epstein pearls on the side of the hard palate
    B. the 2-day-old neonate with apnea lasting 10 seconds
    C. the 24-hour-old neonate who has nasal flaring
    D. the 2-hour-old neonate with a bluish white, moist umbilical cord with one vein and two arteries visible

23. Match the term with its description.

    A. anal patency   _____   Touching cheek along the side of the mouth causes infant to turn head
                                      toward the side and begin to suck.
    B. Down syndrome
                             _____   fanning of the toes and dorsiflexion of the great toe; found in infants until
    C. rooting reflex   about 24 months of age

    D. Babinski   _____   symmetric abduction and extension of the arms, fingers fan out, and thumb
                                      and index finger form a C
    E. Moro reflex
                             _____   passage of meconium during first 48 hours of life
    F. tonic neck
                             _____   transverse palmar crease

                             _____   Infant in supine position turns head to one side with jaw over shoulder,
                                      with extension of the arm and leg on the side to which the head is turned
                                      and flexion of the opposite side.

24. At birth the major cause of heat loss is by:
    A. evaporation.
    B. radiation.
    C. conduction.
    D. convection.

25. The nurse implements all of the following actions to maintain a patent airway in a newborn. Which one will be LEAST effective?
    A. maintaining the healthy infant in a supine or side-lying position during sleep
    B. maintaining the infant with breathing problems in a prone position during sleep
    C. when suctioning the infant in the delivery room, suctioning the pharynx first, then the nasal passages
    D. continuing oral feedings for the infant with nasal flaring and intercostal retractions

26. Identify the correct medication to be given to provide prevention care.

    _____ A. prophylactic eye treatment against ophthalmia neonatorum

    _____ B. administered by injection to prevent hemorrhagic disease of the newborn

    _____ C. first dose given between birth and 2 days of age to decrease incidence of HBV

27. The nurse should involve the parents in the care of their newborn. Teaching is LEAST likely to include:
    A. the use of Ivory soap, oils, powder, and lotions with each bath.
    B. cleaning of the vulva by a front-to-back direction or cleaning of the foreskin by wiping around the glans. If the foreskin is retracted, it must be by gentle retraction only as far as it will go, with gentle return to normal position as necessary. The foreskin is not retracted in the newborn because it is normally tight.
    C. care of the umbilical stump, including placing the diaper below the cord to avoid irritation and wetness of the site.
    D. care of the circumcision site if necessary to include the fact that on the second day a yellowish white exudate forms normally as part of the granulating process.

28. Human milk is preferable to cow's milk because:
    A. human milk has a non-laxative effect.
    B. human milk has more calories per ounce.
    C. human milk has greater mineral content.
    D. human milk offers greater immunologic benefits.

29. The nurse is instructing new parents about proper feeding techniques for their newborns. Identify the following statements as either TRUE or FALSE.

    _____ Infants need at least two hours of sucking daily.

    _____ After feeding, infants should be placed on the right side to prevent regurgitation and distention.

    _____ Breast-fed infants tend to be hungry every two to three hours.

    _____ Supplemental feedings should not be offered to the breast-fed infant because they cause nipple confusion.

    _____ Supplemental water is not needed in breast-fed infants, even in hot climates.

    _____ Five behavioral stages occur during successful feeding. These are prefeeding, approach, attachment, consummatory, and satiety behaviors.

30. Which one of the following actions by the nurse will be LEAST likely to promote the attachment process of the infant and parent?
    A. recognizing individual differences present in the infant and explaining these normal characteristics to the parent
    B. assisting the mother to assume the en face position when she is presented with her infant
    C. explaining to the parents how to react to their infant with the use of reciprocal interacting
    D. explaining to the parents the need for infants to have an organized schedule of daily activities which allows the infant to remain in his/her crib during awake periods

❖ *Critical Thinking* ❖
Case Study

Michael was born by normal vaginal delivery to Marilyn and Doug Madison. His Apgar score at 1 minute was 9 and his Apgar score at 5 minutes was 10. His weight was 6 pounds and his length was 21 inches. Mrs. Madison was allowed to hold Michael and put him to breast in the delivery room. The Madisons do not plan on circumcision for Michael.

31. Listed below are nursing actions that the nurse would perform during the transitional period. List these actions in order of priority.
    1. taking head and chest circumference measurements
    2. assessing for neonatal distress
    3. administering prophylactic medications
    4. scoring for gestational age
    5. assessing vital signs
    A. 2, 5, 1, 3, 4
    B. 1, 2, 5, 3, 4
    C. 2, 3, 1, 5, 4
    D. 2, 5, 4, 1, 3

32. Identify four goals for Michael in order of priority.

    _____

    _____

    _____

    _____

33. You are assigned to care for Michael in the newborn nursery. Michael is now 1 day old. List daily assessments that the nurse recognizes should be conducted and documented.

    _____

    _____

    _____

    _____

    _____

    _____

34. Mrs. Madison and Michael are being discharged tomorrow. You are preparing to provide Mrs. Madison with the newborn discharge teaching plan. Michael is Mrs. Madison's first infant, and on assessment you find that Mrs. Madison has several questions about her techniques of breast-feeding. You show Mrs. Madison how to hold Michael for feeding, how to properly position him to facilitate sucking, and how to care for her breast; and you provide her with a video to reinforce your instruction. When you return later, Mrs. Madison asks you about the use of supplemental feedings. Your best response would be:
   A. "It is okay to give Michael supplements but only after he is put to the breast."
   B. "Why would you think about that now? We'll discuss it tomorrow when you are ready to go home."
   C. "There is no need to give Michael supplemental feedings. Supplemental feeding can cause nipple confusion and decrease milk production."
   D. "You will need to give Michael supplemental feedings sometimes because you may not have enough milk."

35. The nurse correctly evaluates her teaching plan as effective when:
   A. Mrs. Madison is discharged to take Michael home.
   B. Mrs. Madison explains to the nurse how to successfully breast-feed Michael.
   C. Mrs. Madison is observed by the nurse to successfully breast-feed Michael. Additionally, Mrs. Madison discusses with the nurse the information the nurse previously shared with her on breast-feeding.
   D. Mrs. Madison verbalizes that she has no further questions about breast-feeding and is able to describe to the nurse the teaching that was provided.

❖ Crossword Puzzle ❖

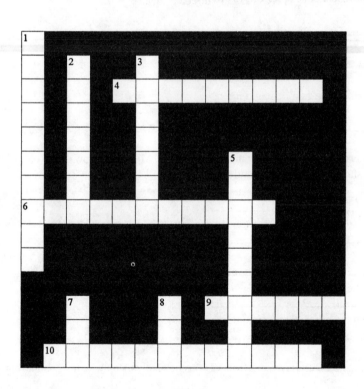

Across

4. Woman who has had two or more pregnancies that resulted in viable fetuses
6. Development of paternal attachment to infant
9. Referring to the top of the head
10. Removal of the foreskin on the glans penis

Down

1. Emotional development from infant to parent
2. Brazelton Neonatal Behavioral Assessment Scale
3. Bands of connective tissue between cranial bones
5. Spaces of unossified membranous tissue located on the cranium
7. Neonatal Perception Inventory
8. Absorbent gelling material

❖ CHAPTER 9
Health Problems of the Newborn

1. Birth injuries may occur during the delivery of the infant. Birth injuries are NOT usually the result of:
   A. forceful extraction delivery.
   B. dystocia.
   C. excessive amniotic fluid.
   D. breech presentation.

2. Which one of the following soft tissue birth injuries is MOST likely to need further evaluation?
   A. subcutaneous fat necrosis
   B. ecchymoses
   C. petechiae appearing in areas other than the presenting part
   D. petechiae appearing on the presenting part

3. Nursing care for soft tissue injury is NOT usually directed toward:
   A. assessing the injury.
   B. preventing breakdown and infection.
   C. providing explanation and reassurance to the parents.
   D. explaining the need for careful follow-up of injury after the infant's discharge.

4. Match the type of extracranial hemorrhagic injury with its description.

   A. caput succedaneum   _____   bleeding into the area between the periosteum and bone; does not cross the suture line

   B. subgaleal hemorrhage

                                     _____   bleeding into the potential space that contains loosely arranged connective

   C. cephalhematoma   tissue

                                       _____   edematous tissue above the bone; extends across sutures

5. Fracture of the clavicle is the most frequent birth injury. Which one of the following would the nurse expect to observe on the physical examination of this infant?
   A. crepitus felt over the affected area
   B. symmetrical Moro reflex
   C. complete fracture with overriding fragments
   D. totally absent Moro reflex

6. Match the type of paralysis with its description. (Types of paralysis may be used more than once.)

   A. facial paralysis   _____   arm hangs limp with the shoulder and arm adducted and internally rotated

   B. brachial palsy

                                       _____   inability to close the eye completely on the affected side with loss

   C. phrenic nerve paralysis   of movement on the affected side; drooping of the corner of the mouth and absence of forehead wrinkling

                                       _____   usually spontaneously disappears in a few days but may take several months

_____ causes diaphragmatic paralysis with respiratory distress the most common sign of injury; usually unilateral injury with affected side lung not expanding

_____ Nursing care includes maintaining proper positioning and preventing contractures.

_____ Nursing care is aimed at aiding the infant in sucking and the mother with feeding techniques.

_____ Undressing begins with the unaffected side, while dressing begins with the affected side.

_____ Artificial tears are instilled to prevent drying.

7. Which one of the following does the nurse recognize as NOT being correct in describing erythema toxicum neonatorum?
A. It is a benign, self-limiting rash that appears within the first 2 days of life.
B. The rash is most obvious during crying episodes.
C. The rash may be located on all areas of the body including the soles of the feet and the palms of the hands.
D. Lesions appear as 1- to 3-mm, white or pale yellow pustules with an erythematous base. Smears of the pustules show increased numbers of eosinophils and lowered numbers of neutrophils.

8. The nurse is preparing to teach a class to new parents about candidiasis. In organizing her presentation, which of the following statements does the nurse recognize as TRUE and which as FALSE?

_____ Candidiasis is a yeast-like fungus that can be transmitted by maternal vaginal infection during delivery, by person-to-person contact, and from contaminated articles.

_____ In the neonate, candidiasis is usually found in the oral and diaper areas.

_____ It is difficult to distinguish between oral candidiasis and coagulated milk in the infant's mouth because both are easily removed by simple wiping.

_____ Candidal dermatitis exists best in the warm, moist atmosphere found in the diaper.

_____ Candidal dermatitis is treated by administration of oral nystatin four times a day after meals.

_____ The infant can spread candidal dermatitis into the mouth with contaminated hands; therefore, the parents should be taught to place clothes over the diaper to break this cycle.

_____ It is not necessary to boil bottles or nipples for infants with oral candidiasis because the fungus is heat-resistant.

_____ Warm saline compresses are applied to the lesions before each diaper change.

9. Which one of the following is NOT a correct description of impetigo and should be omitted by the nurse from the teaching plan?
A. Impetigo is caused by _Staphylococcus aureus_.
B. Impetigo is an eruption of vesicular lesions that occur on skin that has not been traumatized.
C. Distribution of the lesions usually occurs on the perineum, trunk, face, and buttocks.
D. Impetigo requires that the infected child or infant be isolated from others until all lesions have healed.

10. Label the following statements with the correct birthmark identification.

_____ These lesions are pink, red, or purple and often thicken, darken, and pro-
portionately enlarge as the child grows.

_____ These are red, rubbery nodules with a rough surface which are recognized
as tumors that involve only capillaries.

11. Hyperbilirubinemia is an excessive accumulation of bilirubin in the blood and is characterized by

_____, a yellow discoloration of the skin.

12. In discussing the pathophysiology of bilirubin, the nurse knows that red blood cell destruction results in

_____ and _____. _____ _____ is an

insoluble substance. In the liver this is changed to a soluble substance, _____ _____.

13. What is the term used to describe the yellow staining of the brain cells that can result in bilirubin encephalopathy?
A. jaundice
B. physiologic jaundice
C. kernicterus
D. icterus neonatorum

14. Which one of the following statements about bilirubin encephalopathy is TRUE?
A. Development may be enhanced by metabolic acidosis, lowered albumin levels, free fatty acids, and certain drugs
such as sulfonamides.
B. It produces no permanent neurologic damage.
C. Serum bilirubin levels alone can predict the risk of brain injury.
D. It produces permanent liver damage by deposits of conjugated bilirubin within the cell.

15. A newborn developed jaundice at 48 hours' age that peaked at 72 hours and declined at about age 7 days. The MOST
likely cause of this hyperbilirubinemia is:
A. physiologic jaundice.
B. pathologic jaundice.
C. hemolytic disease of the newborn.
D. ABO blood incompatibility.

16. Of the four infants listed below, which one would the nurse recognize as being LEAST likely to develop jaundice?
A. an infant with subgaleal hemorrhage which is now resolving
B. an infant with cephalhematoma which is now resolving
C. the infant who has feedings started early, which will stimulate peristalsis and rapid passage of meconium
D. the infant who is of Native American descent

17. Therapy differs between breast-feeding-associated jaundice and breast milk jaundice. Which one of the following
would the nurse expect to implement with breast milk jaundice?
A. Increase frequency of breast-feedings.
B. Permanently discontinue breast-feedings.
C. Discontinue breast-feedings for no more than 24 hours.
D. Increase frequency of breast-feedings and add caloric supplements.

18. Newborns are more prone to produce higher levels of bilirubin because they:
    1. have a higher concentration of circulating erythrocytes.
    2. have red blood cells with a shorter life span.
    3. have reduced albumin concentrations.
    4. have an anatomically underdeveloped liver.
    A. 1, 2, 3, and 4
    B. 1, 2, and 3
    C. 2, 3, and 4
    D. 3 and 4

19. Which of the following is TRUE regarding diagnostic evaluations for bilirubin?
    A. Newborn levels of unconjugated bilirubin usually must exceed 5 mg/dl before jaundice is observable.
    B. Hyperbilirubinemia is defined as a serum bilirubin value of 8 mg/dl in full-term infants.
    C. When jaundice occurs before the infant is 24 hours of age, bilirubin level assessment is unnecessary.
    D. Transcutaneous bilirubinometry is an effective cutaneous measurement of bilirubin in full-term infants being treated with phototherapy.

20. Phototherapy is the usual form of treatment for hyperbilirubinemia. Which one of the following does the nurse NOT include in the plan of care for an infant receiving phototherapy?
    A. The infant's eyes will be shielded by an opaque mask to prevent exposure to the light.
    B. Once phototherapy has been started, visual assessment of jaundice increases in validity; therefore, fewer serum bilirubin levels will be necessary.
    C. charting of the phototherapy to include the time it was started and stopped, the manufacturer of the fluorescent lamp, the number of lamps, and the photometer measurement of light intensity
    D. assessment of the infant for side effects to include loose, greenish stools, skin rashes, hyperthermia, dehydration, and increased metabolic rate

21. Fill in the blanks in the following statements.

    A. Erythroblastosis fetalis is caused by _____ _____.

    B. The nurse is reviewing maternal hematologic laboratory results. The nurse knows that the _____

    _____ is the test that monitors anti-Rh antibody titers. The test performed postnatally to detect

    maternal antibodies attached to the circulating erythrocytes of affected infants is called _____

    _____.

    C. In order to be effective in preventing maternal sensitization to the Rh factor, the nurse must administer Rho immune

    globulin (RhoGam) within _____ _____ after the first delivery or abortion

    and with each subsequent pregnancy. RhoGam is administered to the _____

    _____ _____ by the _____ route.

22. In the full-term neonate, which one of the following fits the definition of hypoglycemia? Plasma glucose concentrations of:
    A. less than 50 mg/dl at 48 hours of age.
    B. less than 60 mg/dl at 48 hours of age.
    C. less than 40 mg/dl at 25 hours of age.
    D. less than 60 mg/dl at birth.

23. What assessment finding is the nurse MOST likely to see in the infant as a result of hypoglycemia?
    A. forceful, low-pitched cry
    B. tachypnea
    C. jitteriness, tremors, twitching
    D. vomiting, refusal to eat

24. The nurse caring for the infant with hypocalcemia recognizes that which one of the following is included in the care plan?
    A. Scalp veins are the preferred site for intravenous administration of calcium gluconate.
    B. Signs of hypercalcemia include vomiting and bradycardia.
    C. Stimuli should be increased until calcium levels rise.
    D. Calcium gluconate is compatible with sodium bicarbonate.

25. The nurse is assessing Sarah, a neonate born at home two days ago, and observes blood oozing from the umbilicus. What is the MOST likely cause of Sarah's hemorrhagic disease?
    A. The neonate is born with an anatomically immature liver.
    B. Coagulation factors (II, VII, IX, X) are deactivated in the neonate.
    C. administration of vitamin K to the neonate shortly after birth
    D. The newborn is born with a sterile intestine and is unable to synthesize vitamin K until feedings are begun.

26. When teaching the parents of the newborn about testing for PKU, the nurse should include which one of the following key points?
    A. The test is performed only on infants expected to have the disorder.
    B. The test is performed on cord blood.
    C. The test is not reliable if the blood sample is taken after the infant has ingested a source of protein.
    D. The test should be performed on all newborns before they leave the hospital, and a repeat blood specimen should be obtained by the third week of life if the first test was taken within the first 24 hours of life.

27. In educating the parents of a newborn with galactosemia, the nurse includes which one of the following in the plan?
    A. All food labels should be read carefully for the presence of lactose.
    B. Once the diagnosis is made and the diet is altered, little follow-up of these infants is necessary.
    C. Breast milk is acceptable for infants with galactosemia.
    D. Signs of visual impairment are unlikely in children with this disorder.

28. Treatment for congenital hypothyroidism involves lifelong thyroid hormone replacement. The drug of choice is

_____.

❖ Critical Thinking ❖
Case Study

Mrs. Becker had a normal pregnancy and delivery without complications at 39 weeks' gestation. She is breast-feeding her 2-day-old neonate, Ben, when she notices that his skin looks yellow. The total serum bilirubin level is 13 mg/dl.

29. Mrs. Becker asks the nurse about Ben's condition and the seriousness of his illness. Which one of the following is the BEST response?
    A. "Ben has pathologic jaundice, a serious condition."
    B. "Ben has breast milk jaundice, and you will need to permanently stop breast-feeding."
    C. "Ben has physiologic jaundice, a normal finding at his age."
    D. "Infants with serum bilirubin levels of 13 mg/dl will develop bilirubin encephalopathy and severe brain damage."

30. The physician orders that Mrs. Becker increase her frequency of breast-feeding to every two hours and avoid supplementation. The rationale for this management is being discussed by the nurse with Mrs. Becker. Which one of the following does the nurse recognize as the basis for the ordered treatment?
    A. The jaundice is related to the process of breast-feeding, probably from decreased caloric and fluid intake by breast-fed infants.
    B. The jaundice is caused by a factor in the breast milk that breaks down bilirubin to a lipid-soluble form, which is reabsorbed in the gut.
    C. The jaundice is caused by the mother's hemolytic disease.
    D. The jaundice is increased because the infant was put to breast early, which increases the amount of time meconium is kept in the gut before excretion.

31. The serum bilirubin level has not decreased as desired and phototherapy has been ordered. The priority goal at this time is:
    A. the infant will be evaluated for neurological deficit.
    B. the infant will receive adequate intravenous hydration.
    C. the infant will experience no complications from phototherapy.
    D. the infant will experience no complications from exchange transfusion.

32. When caring for Ben the nurse should take all but which of the following actions to prevent complications?
    A. Make certain that eyelids are closed before applying eye shields. Check eyes at least every shift for discharge or irritation.
    B. Monitor axillary temperature closely to detect hyperthermia and/or hypothermia.
    C. Maintain 18 inches' distance between infant and light.
    D. Apply oil daily to skin to avoid breakdown.

33. An expected patient outcome for Ben while on phototherapy is:
    A. newborn begins feeding soon after birth.
    B. family demonstrates an understanding of therapy and prognosis.
    C. ensure adequate intake to prevent dehydration.
    D. newborn displays no evidence of eye irritation, dehydration, temperature instability, or skin breakdown.

❖ Crossword Puzzle ❖

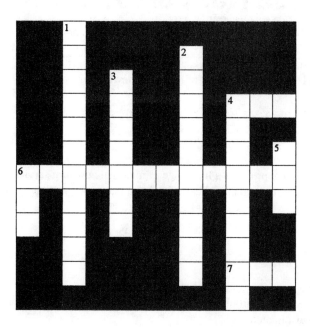

Across

4. Hemolytic disease of the newborn
6. Having dissimilar genes at a given position on a pair of chromosomes
7. Inborn error of metabolism

Down

1. Toxic accumulation of bilirubin in central nervous system tissue
2. Having the same genes at a given position on a pair of chromosomes
3. Jaundice
4. Related to destruction of red blood cells
5. Thyroid-stimulating hormone
6. Hemoglobin

❖ CHAPTER 10
The High-Risk Newborn and Family

1. Which one of the following is NOT a classification of high-risk newborns?
   A. according to birth size
   B. according to gestational age
   C. according to mortality
   D. according to birth age

2. A neonatal intensive care facility that provides a full range of maternal newborn services and that has the capacity to provide care for the most complex neonatal complications with at least one full-time neonatologist on staff is known as a:
   A. Level I facility.
   B. Level II facility.
   C. Level III facility.
   D. Level IV facility.

3. When the high-risk neonate needs transportation to a facility that can provide intensive care, the nurse recognizes that priority care for this neonate must include:
   A. transfer of both the mother and infant.
   B. immediate transport, often before stabilization of the neonate.
   C. delay of transport until the neonate has been sufficiently stabilized for transport.
   D. a transport team composed of at least a neonatologist, a respiratory therapist, and one neonatal nurse.

4. A thorough systematic physical assessment is a must in the care of the high-risk neonate. Subtle changes in

   _____ _____, _____, _____, or

   _____ _____ often indicate an underlying problem.

5. At birth the newborn is immediately assessed to determine any apparent problems and to identify those that demand immediate attention. The assessment NOT normally conducted at birth or immediately after birth is:
   A. assignment of a gestational age score.
   B. assignment of an Apgar score.
   C. evaluation for obvious congenital anomalies.
   D. evaluation for neonatal distress.

6. Identify the following statements about high-risk care of the neonate as either TRUE or FALSE.

   _____ Neonates under intensive observation are placed in a controlled environment and monitored for heart rate, respiratory activity, and temperature.

   _____ Sophisticated monitoring and life-support systems can replace the observations of the infant by nursing personnel.

   _____ Electrodes for cardiac monitors should not be applied to the back or upper arms of the neonate.

   _____ Infants who are mechanically ventilated and have low Apgar scores can have lower blood pressures.

_____ An accurate output can be obtained in the neonate by use of a urine collecting bag or by weighing the infant's diaper. Regardless of the method utilized, 40 gram weight of urine would be recorded as 40 ml of urine.

_____ The nurse is preparing the infant for a heel stick. This is done to create adequate vasodilation and is accomplished by placing a heating pad on the infant's heel.

_____ Nurses are allowed to turn off alarm systems for electronic monitoring devices when their sounds disturb the infant's parents.

7. The major source of increased heat production during cold stress in the high-risk neonate is _____

   _____.

8. Low-birth-weight infants are at a disadvantage for heat production compared with full-term infants because they have:
   1. small muscle mass.
   2. fewer deposits of brown fat.
   3. less insulating subcutaneous fat.
   4. poor reflex control of skin capillaries.
   A. 1, 2, 3, and 4
   B. 2, 3, and 4
   C. 1, 2, and 3
   D. 1, 3, and 4

9. Cold stress produces three major consequences that pose additional hazards to the neonate. These are:

   _____

   _____

   _____

10. The nurse recognizes an intervention LEAST likely to be effective for the high-risk neonate as which one of the following?
    A. maintaining a neutral thermal environment
    B. placing the heat-sensing probe on the infant's abdomen when the infant is in the prone position
    C. keeping oxygen that is supplied to the infant via a hood around the head warmed and humidified
    D. warming all items that come in direct contact with the infant including the hands of caregivers

11. The BEST way to prevent infection in the high-risk neonate begins with:
    A. meticulous and frequent handwashing of all persons coming in contact with the infant.
    B. observing continually for signs of infection.
    C. requiring everyone working in the NICU to put on fresh scrub clothes before entering the unit.
    D. performing epidemiologic studies at least monthly.

12. A complication that develops with the use of an umbilical catheter is thrombi. The nurse recognizes this complication because of the appearance of:
    A. increased warmth in lower extremities.
    B. bluish discoloration seen in the toes, called "cath toes."
    C. inability of the kidneys to produce urine.
    D. hemorrhage from the umbilical catheter area.

13. What is the BEST indication that the preterm infant can tolerate nipple feedings?
    A. The infant requires approximately 40 minutes to complete a feeding.
    B. The infant has a sustained respiratory rate of 68.
    C. The infant is able to suck on a pacifier.
    D. The infant has a coordinated suck-swallow reflex.

14. The physician has directed the nurse to begin gavage feeding for an infant who weighs less than 1500 g. The nurse includes which one of the following in the implementation of gavage feedings?
    A. Insert the tube into the unobstructed nares.
    B. Perform the procedure with the infant in a supine position with the head elevated 45 degrees.
    C. Aspirate the contents of the stomach, measure these contents, and replace the residual before beginning the feeding. The amount of residual is subtracted from the total feeding to prevent over-distending the stomach.
    D. Allow the feeding to flow by gravity, then push a small amount of the feeding into the stomach, then allow the remainder of the feeding to flow by gravity.

15. _____ _____ increases oxygenation during tube feeding and has been shown to increase readiness in low-birth-weight infants for bottle-feeding.

16. One of the major goals of care for the high-risk neonate is conservation of energy. This is LEAST likely accomplished by which of the following actions?
    A. organizing nursing care activities so that the infant is not overstimulated and not overdisturbed
    B. maintaining a neutral thermal environment
    C. keeping the infant in the supine position as much as possible to decrease expenditure of energy by unnecessary movement
    D. employing gavage feeding

17. In caring for preterm infants the nurse knows to:
    A. use scissors to remove dressings or tape from the infant's extremities.
    B. use solvents to remove tape from the neonate's delicate skin.
    C. avoid use of bland, nonalkaline soaps in removal of stool.
    D. use transparent elastic film dressings to secure and protect central lines.

18. Promoting a healthy parent-child relationship for the family with a high-risk neonate is BEST accomplished by the nurse:
    A. reinforcing parents' involvement during caregiving activities and interactions with their infant.
    B. providing guidance to parents in their efforts to meet their infant's needs.
    C. allowing the parents to express feelings of helplessness and lack of control.
    D. providing support during the initial visit with their infant.

19. The term _____ _____ _____ is applied to physically healthy children who are perceived by the parents to be at high risk for medical or developmental problems.

20. Discharge instructions for the parents of the preterm infant should NOT include:
    A. warning parents that their infant may still be in danger and will need constant attention.
    B. providing information to the parents on how to contact personnel for questions after discharge.
    C. instructions about car safety seats including how these seats can be adapted for smaller children with the placement of blanket rolls on each side of the infant to support the head and trunk.
    D. providing adequate information about immunization needs.

21. A physical characteristic usually observed in the preterm infant and NOT observed in the full-term infant is:
    A. a proportionately equal head in relation to the body.
    B. skin that is often translucent, smooth, and shiny with small blood vessels clearly visible underneath the epidermis.
    C. soles of feet and palms of hand with distinct creases extending across the entire palms and down the complete soles of the feet.
    D. absence of lanugo and little vernix caseosa.

22. Post-term or postmature infants are:
    A. infants born with a gestation equal to 38 weeks.
    B. infants born before 41 weeks of gestation.
    C. infants born of a gestation that extends beyond 42 weeks as calculated from the mother's last menstrual period.
    D. infants born of a gestation that extends beyond 43 weeks as calculated from the mother's last menstrual period.

23. Apnea in the preterm infant is defined as a lapse of spontaneous breathing lasting for how many seconds?
    A. 5
    B. 10
    C. 15
    D. 20

24. Bryan is a 2-day-old preterm infant being cared for in the NICU. He had some apnea periods, but in report the nurse was told he had had no episodes today. His apnea monitor alarm has just sounded. What is the FIRST action of the nurse?
    A. Use tactile stimulation, rubbing on the back to stop the apneic spell.
    B. Suction the nose and oropharynx.
    C. Assess the infant for color and for presence of respiration.
    D. Shake the infant.

25. A late and serious sign of respiratory distress in the neonate is:
    A. central cyanosis.
    B. respiratory rate of 90 breaths/minute.
    C. substernal retractions.
    D. nasal flaring.

26. Preterm infants who have high blood oxygen levels from exposure to prolonged oxygen therapy are at risk for developing:
    A. retinopathy of prematurity.
    B. cataracts.
    C. pneumothorax.
    D. tracheal perforation.

27. Susie, a 20-minute-old neonate, was observed at birth to have meconium staining. If Susie has meconium in the lungs, this presence will:
    A. prevent air from entering the lungs.
    B. trap inspired air in the lungs.
    C. increase the production of surfactant.
    D. lead to respiratory alkalosis.

28. An important nursing function is close observation for neonates at risk for developing air leaks. These infants include:
    A. infants with respiratory distress syndrome (RDS).
    B. infants with meconium-stained amniotic fluid.
    C. infants receiving CPAP or positive-pressure ventilation.
    D. all of the above.

29. Infants diagnosed with bronchopulmonary dyplasia have special care needs. These needs include:
    A. opportunities for adequate rest.
    B. increases in environmental stimuli.
    C. decreases in caloric intake.
    D. rapid weaning from ventilators.

30. The laboratory evaluation for the diagnosis of sepsis is LEAST likely to include:
    A. blood cultures.
    B. spinal fluid culture.
    C. urine culture.
    D. gastric secretion culture.

31. Clinical signs seen in necrotizing enterocolitis are:
    A. increased abdominal girth.
    B. increased gastric residual.
    C. positive stool hematest.
    D. all of the above.

32. Preterm infants can develop patent ductus arteriosus (PDA). Therapy often includes the administration of:
    A. theophylline.
    B. indomethacin.
    C. digoxin.
    D. heparin.

33. The nurse should carefully monitor and record amounts of all blood drawn for tests in the preterm infant. The reason is:
    A. early detection of anemia.
    B. prevention of infection.
    C. prevention of polycythemia.
    D. hypothermia regulation.

34. The preterm infant is in danger of developing retinopathy of prematurity (ROP). Of the following nursing actions, which one is LEAST likely to be effective in the prevention of ROP?
    A. correct oxygen administration
    B. decreasing environmental stimuli, direct light
    C. avoiding scalp vein intravenous infusion
    D. monitoring of oxygenation status

35. The nurse recognizes that which of the following interventions is CONTRAINDICATED in the preterm infant with increased intracranial pressure?
    A. avoiding interventions that produce crying
    B. administering blood/blood products
    C. administering analgesics to reduce discomfort
    D. turning the head to the right without body alignment

36. The nurse is able to distinguish between seizures and jitteriness in the neonate. Identify which one of the following is NOT a description of seizures.
    A. Seizures are not accompanied by ocular movement.
    B. Seizures have their dominant movement as tremor.
    C. In seizures the dominant movement cannot be stopped by flexion of the affected limb.
    D. Seizures are highly sensitive to light manual stimulation.

37. John is a newborn just delivered of a diabetic mother. The nurse will watch John for signs that he is rapidly developing what?
    A. hyperglycemia
    B. hypoglycemia
    C. pancreatic failure
    D. dehydration

38. Infants born to narcotic-addicted mothers will exhibit all of the following clinical manifestations EXCEPT:
    A. tremors and restlessness.
    B. frequent sneezing.
    C. coordinated suck and swallow reflex.
    D. high-pitched, shrill cry.

❖ Critical Thinking ❖
Case Study

Baby Mark was born at 36 weeks' gestation and weighed 2300 g at birth. Apgar score at 1 minute was 5. Baby Mark was suctioned and oxygen administration started. He responded with spontaneous respirations. You are the nurse who has been assigned to care for him in the special care nursery. Mark's admission vital signs are pulse 150, respirations 56, and axillary temperature 96.4° F. Mark is placed in a radiant warmer and oxygen continued by oxygen hood.

39. You would classify Baby Mark as:
    1. full-term.
    2. preterm.
    3. low birth weight.
    4. small for gestational age.
    A. 1 and 4
    B. 2 and 4
    C. 2 and 3
    D. 1 and 3

40. You identify Mark as being at risk for developing respiratory distress syndrome. Why?
    1. gestational age
    2. low Apgar score
    3. hypothermia
    4. respiratory rate of 56
    A. 1, 2, 3, and 4
    B. 1, 2, and 3
    C. 2, 3, and 4
    D. 2 and 3

41. The nurse's plan for oxygen administration includes:
    A. frequent suctioning.
    B. frequent assessment to include unobstructed nares.
    C. nipple feeding with respiratory rates of 70 and below.
    D. turning off monitor alarms to allow the neonate to rest.

42. Baby Mark's parents are visiting him for the first time. How can the nurse assist the parents in feeling more comfortable in the NICU atmosphere?
    A. Discourage questions of a technical nature.
    B. Tell the parents that Mark is going to be fine.
    C. Explain what is happening with Mark and why he is receiving this type of care.
    D. Leave the parents alone with the infant.

43. The nurse will develop a plan of care for Mark that recognizes which of the following as the BEST expected outcome?
    A. Oxygen is administered correctly, and arterial blood gases are within normal limits.
    B. Maintain neutral thermal environment.
    C. Record oxygen delivery rates every two hours.
    D. Assess respiratory status every hour.

❖ Crossword Puzzle ❖

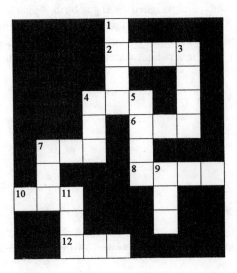

Across

2. Continuous positive airway pressure
4. Apnea of prematurity
6. Peak inspiratory pressure
7. Patent ductus arteriosus
8. Neonatal intensive care unit
10. Intracranial pressure
12. Retinopathy of prematurity

Down

1. Extracorporeal membrane oxygenation
3. Positive end-expiratory pressure
4. Appropriate for gestational age
5. Persistent pulmonary hypertension of the newborn
7. Persistent fetal circulation
9. Infant of diabetic mother
11. Pulmonary vascular resistance

❖ CHAPTER 11
Conditions Caused by Defects in Physical Development

1. Match the term with its description.

   A. growth

   B. hyperplasia

   C. hypertrophy

   D. differentiation

   E. organogenesis

   F. teratogenesis

   G. sensitive or critical periods

   _____ prenatal growth process disturbed to produce a structural or functional defect

   _____ major impact of environmental factors coincides with this period

   _____ beginning of all major organ systems

   _____ cells divide and synthesize new proteins

   _____ increase in cell number

   _____ increase in cell size

   _____ early cells modified and specialized to form the individual

2. Parental responses to the birth of an infant with a physical disability are BEST described as:
   A. hostility and bitterness.
   B. disbelief and denial.
   C. strengthening of the psychologic attachment the mother has formed during pregnancy with the unborn child.
   D. establishment of realistic goals.

3. The nurse can independently implement which one of the following actions in the preoperative neonate?
   A. Start a peripheral intravenous line.
   B. Begin administration of prophylactic antibiotics.
   C. Provide accurate information to the newborn's parents regarding what to expect postoperatively.
   D. Begin pain management control.

4. Primary roles of the nurse in the care of an infant born with a physical defect are:
   A. provider of parental support during the grief process by helping to facilitate the formation of a satisfactory adjustment to the child.
   B. role of caregiver to the infant and to support and encourage the parents in their caregiving tasks.
   C. supplier of information to parents by giving accurate, up-to-date information in language the parents can understand.
   D. all of the above.

5. Identify the following statements about postoperative care of the neonate as either TRUE or FALSE.

   _____ The newborn's poor chest wall stability, along with smaller and more reactive airways, contributes to postoperative respiratory compromise.

   _____ Most postoperative neonates require mechanical ventilation.

   _____ Neonates are highly subject to acidosis and hypoxia and require continuous monitoring of acid-base balance and oxygen status.

_____ The preterm infant is at high risk for developing respiratory complications from general anesthesia.

_____ The neonate is particularly sensitive to vagal stimulation which can be induced by postoperative naso-gastric tubes, endotracheal tubes, and suctioning.

_____ The neonate's risk for rapid fluid shifts can be intensified by stress and loss of fluid during surgical procedures.

6. Manifestations of acute pain in the neonate include:
   A. cardiorespiratory changes, which include increases in heart rate and blood pressure.
   B. hyperglycemia.
   C. increased wakefulness and irritability.
   D. all of the above.

7. A. _____ is the most widely used narcotic analgesic for pharmacologic management of neonatal pain.

   B. List at least three nonpharmacologic measures that can be used by the nurse in the NICU to reduce discomfort in the neonate.

   _____

   _____

   _____

8. Research has shown that supplemental folic acid can reduce the recurrence rates of spina bifida, anencephaly, and encephalocele. How should this supplement be administered?
   A. daily folic acid dose of 4.0 mg beginning 1 month before conception and during the first trimester
   B. daily folic acid dose of 0.4 mg as soon as pregnancy is confirmed
   C. daily folic acid dose of 4.0 mg given through the use of multivitamin preparations beginning 1 month before conception and throughout the first trimester
   D. daily folic acid dose of 4.0 mg beginning with the confirmation of pregnancy and continuing throughout pregnancy

9. Match the medical condition with its description.

   A. anencephaly   _____   failure of neural tube to close and fuse

   B. myelodysplasia   _____   results from disturbances in the dynamics of CSF absorption and flow

   C. myelomeningocele   _____   congenital malformation where both cerebral hemispheres are absent

   D. hydrocephalus   _____   any malformation of the spinal canal and cord

10. The major complications of myelomeningocele are _____ _____

    _____ and _____.

11. Therapeutic management that provides the most favorable (morbidity and mortality) outcome for the child born with myelomeningocele is:
    A. early physical therapy.
    B. closure of the defect within first 24 hours.
    C. prevention of infection.
    D. splint application to lower extremities.

12. Myelomeningocele may be associated with hydrocephalus. What should the nurse assess to identify an infant with hydrocephalus?
    A. upward eye slanting
    B. constant dribbling of urine
    C. wide or bulging fontanels
    D. decreased head circumference

13. Upon delivery of an infant with myelomeningocele, which one of the following nursing actions may be CONTRA-INDICATED?
    A. Examine the membranous cyst for intactness.
    B. Diaper the infant.
    C. Keep moist sterile normal saline dressings on defect.
    D. Keep infant in the prone position.

14. An infant born with spina bifida who needs intermittent urinary catheterization has developed sneezing, wheezing, and a rash over his lower pelvic and genital area. The nurse would suspect this infant has developed:
    A. asthma.
    B. emphysema.
    C. latex allergy.
    D. anaphylaxis.

15. Hydrocephalus that is a result of maldevelopment or an intrauterine infection is called _____.

    Hydrocephalus that is caused by infection, neoplasm, or hemorrhage is called _____.

16. Surgical shunts are often required to provide drainage in the treatment of hydrocephalus. Identify the preferred shunt for infants.
    A. ventriculoperitoneal shunt
    B. ventriculoatrial shunt
    C. ventricular bypass
    D. ventriculopleural shunt

17. The nurse recognizes that which one of the following would be included in the postoperative care of a client with a shunt?
    A. positioning the patient in a head-down position
    B. pumping the shunt to assess function
    C. monitoring for abdominal or peritoneal distention
    D. positioning the child on the side of the operative site to facilitate drainage

18. Posterior fontanel is closed by age _____. Anterior fontanel is closed by age

    _____. Sutures are unable to be separated by ICP by age _____.

19. Identify the following statements about microcephaly as either TRUE or FALSE.

    _____ Microcephaly is defined as a head circumference greater than 5 standard deviations below the mean.

    _____ Primary microcephaly can be caused by irradiation between 4 and 20 weeks of gestation.

    _____ Secondary microcephaly can be caused by infection during the third trimester, the perinatal period, or early infancy.

    _____ All children with microcephaly are mentally retarded.

    _____ There is no treatment for microcephaly.

_____ Nursing care is supportive and directed toward helping parents adjust to a child with cognitive impairment.

20. Therapeutic management for craniosynostosis is:
    A. placement of ventriculoperitoneal shunt.
    B. removal of neoplasm.
    C. release of fused sutures.
    D. supportive assistance for parents.

21. The nurse, in preparing a nursing care plan for the infant born with craniofacial abnormalities, recognizes which of the following as TRUE?
    A. Children with this deformity face erroneous assumptions of mental retardation.
    B. Abnormalities include deformities involving the skull and facial bones.
    C. A helmet is often required after surgery to protect the operative site and bone grafts for six months to two years.
    D. All of the above are true.

22. Match the degree of developmental hip dysplasia with its description.

    A. acetabular dysplasia   _____ Femoral head remains in contact with the acetabulum, but the head of the femur is partially displaced.

    B. subluxation
                                _____ Femoral head remains in the acetabulum (mildest form).

    C. dislocation
                                _____ Femoral head loses contact with the acetabulum.

23. The nurse observes which of the following signs in the infant with developmental hip dysplasia?
    A. positive Ortolani maneuver
    B. asymmetrical folds in skin of legs
    C. shortening of the limb on the affected side
    D. all of the above

24. Match the expected therapeutic management for developmental hip dysplasia with the age group.

    A. newborn to 6 months   _____ more difficult; includes operative reduction and innominate osteotomy procedures designed to construct an acetabular roof

    B. 6 to 18 months
                               _____ abduction devices such as Pavlik harness; can also include skin traction, hip spica cast
    C. older child

                               _____ plaster cast immobilization until stable joint confirmed; individualized home traction may decrease length of hospitalization; open reduction for soft tissue obstruction

25. Match the congenital clubfoot condition with its description.

    A. talipes varus   _____ eversion or bending outward

    B. talipes valgus   _____ inversion or bending inward

    C. talipes equinus   _____ plantar flexion in which the toes are lower then the heel

    D. talipes calcaneus   _____ dorsiflexion, with toes higher than the heel

26. Treatment of clubfoot includes:
    A. manual overcorrection of the deformity.
    B. maintenance of the correction until normal muscle is gained, often accomplished by casts or orthoses.
    C. follow-up observation to detect possible recurrence of the deformity.
    D. all of the above.

27. An important assessment for identifying cleft palate is for the nurse to:
    A. assess sucking ability of infant.
    B. assess color of lips.
    C. palpate the palate with a gloved finger.
    D. all of the above

28. Which of the following is acceptable for feeding the infant with a cleft of the lip or palate?
    1. use of "cleft palate" nipple or large, soft nipple with large hole or breast-feeding
    2. use of normal nipple
    3. use of "gravity flow" nipple attached to a squeezable plastic bottle
    4. use of rubber-tipped asepto syringe or Breck feeder
    A. 1, 2, 3, and 4
    B. 1, 3, and 4
    C. 1, 2, and 4
    D. 1 and 3

29. In providing postoperative care for the infant with a cleft of the lip or palate, which one of the following is CONTRAINDICATED?
    A. elbow restraints applied bilaterally and pinned by the cuffs to the infant's clothes
    B. removal of restraints (only one at a time) at regular intervals for exercise of the arms and inspection of the skin under the restraints
    C. placement of infant in the prone position after cleft lip repair to prevent trauma to the area
    D. placement of the infant in the prone position after cleft palate repair

30. Feeding the infant with a cleft repair of either the lip or the palate postoperatively includes which of the following?
    1. If the infant had cleft lip repair, feeding begins with clear liquid.
    2. Cleft lip repair feedings include use of the Breck feeder. The rubber tip is placed inside from the side of the mouth.
    3. Cleft palate repair feedings include the use of spoons and forks.
    4. Cleft palate repair feedings include the use of cups and straws.
    A. 1 and 2
    B. 1, 2, 3, and 4
    C. 1 and 3
    D. 2 and 4

31. The nurse observes frothy saliva in the mouth and nose of the neonate and frequent drooling. When fed, the infant swallows normally, but suddenly the fluid returns through the nose and mouth of the infant. The nurse would suspect what medical condition?
    A. esophageal atresia
    B. cleft palate
    C. anorectal malformation
    D. biliary atresia

32. The assessment that is MOST likely to indicate absence of anorectal malformation is:
    A. flat perineum.
    B. absence of external sphincter contraction with stimulation.
    C. no difficulty in taking rectal temperature.
    D. passage of meconium stool.

33. The BEST definition of biliary atresia is:
    A. jaundice persisting beyond 2 weeks of age with elevated direct bilirubin levels.
    B. progressive inflammatory process causing intrahepatic and extrahepatic bile duct fibrosis.
    C. absence of bile pigment.
    D. hepatomegaly and palpable liver.

34. Identify the following statements about umbilical hernia as either TRUE or FALSE.

    _____ The disorder affects blacks more than whites.

    _____ It affects preterm infants more than full-term infants.

    _____ It may be present in association with Down syndrome.

    _____ It is most prominent when the infant is crying.

    _____ It usually spontaneously resolves by 3 to 4 years of age.

35. Which one of the following is CONTRAINDICATED as part of the therapeutic management for the neonate with congenital diaphragmatic hernia?
    A. endotracheal intubation
    B. gastrointestinal decompression
    C. positioning the infant with the head and chest elevated above the abdomen
    D. bag and mask ventilation

36. Match the term with its description.

    A. gastroschisis   _____ prevents retraction of the foreskin

    B. omphalocele   _____ herniation of the abdominal contents through the umbilical ring

    C. phimosis   _____ herniation of abdominal contents lateral to the umbilical ring

    D. inguinal hernia   _____ externalization of the bladder

    E. femoral hernia   _____ painless inguinal swelling

    F. cryptorchidism   _____ swelling in the groin area associated with severe pain (most common in females)

    G. hypospadias
                              _____ fluid in the processus vaginalis
    H. epispadias
                              _____ one or both of the testes do not descend
    I. hydrocele
                              _____ urethral opening located below the glans penis or along the ventral surface of penile shaft
    J. bladder exstrophy

                              _____ opening of the urethra on dorsum of penis

37. Identify the following statements as either TRUE or FALSE.

    _____ The infant's anatomy rather than genetic sex is the primary criterion on which the choice of gender should be made.

    _____ TORCH complex is a group of infective agents that cause similar manifestations in the neonate.

_____ A major goal in care of infants suspected of having an infectious disease is identification of the organism.

_____ The teratogenic effect of drugs is not believed to have an effect on the developing fetal tissue until day 15 of gestation.

_____ Behavioral problems, cognitive impairment, and psychosocial deficits can originate from alcohol ingestion by the pregnant mother.

_____ Poor feeding is a characteristic of infants with fetal alcohol syndrome.

❖ Critical Thinking ❖
Case Study

Jane Williams is a newborn diagnosed with myelomeningocele. She has been admitted to the NICU. Initial care for Jane included assessment and prevention of trauma to the protective covering of the myelomeningocele sac.

38. Thirty-six hours after birth, the nurse notes that Jane has developed an elevated temperature, is irritable when touched, and is lethargic. What would the nurse suspect?
    A. hydrocephalus
    B. infection
    C. latex allergy
    D. urinary retention

39. The nursing diagnosis that is MOST relevant is:
    A. altered bowel elimination related to neurological deficits.
    B. high risk for infection related to the presence of infectious organisms.
    C. altered nutrition related to immobility.
    D. altered self-concept related to physical disability.

40. Which one of the following is the BEST way for the infant with unrepaired myelomeningocele to have tactile stimulation needs met?
    A. by frequent cuddling and being held in parent's arms
    B. by having black and white drawings placed within the infant's view
    C. by frequent caressing and stroking while the infant is placed on a pillow across the parent's lap
    D. by frequent changing of the infant's diaper and dressing

41. Jane has corrective surgery and is six hours postoperative. The nurse must observe the abdomen closely for the development of _____ _____.

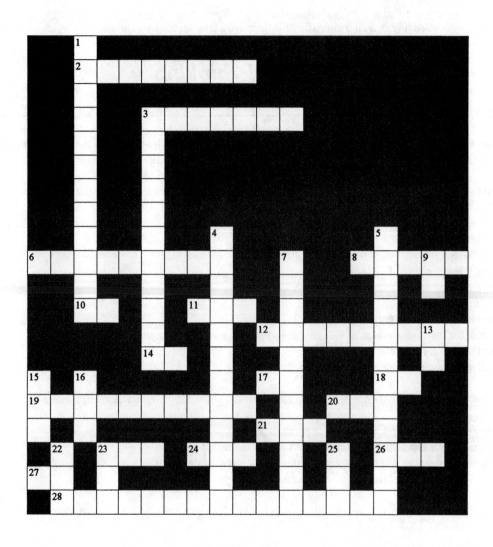

Across

2. Absence of a body part caused by lack of primordial tissue
3. Marked deviation from the normal
6. Abnormal organization of cells into tissue(s) and its morphologic result(s)
8. Toxoplasmosis, other, rubella, CMV, herpes
10. Spina bifida
11. Occipital frontal circumference
12. A substance, agent, or process that interferes with normal prenatal development
14. Nasogastric
17. Cleft palate
18. Esophageal atresia
19. Present at birth
20. Cleft lip and palate
21. Fetal alcohol syndrome
23. Congenital dislocated hip
24. Clean intermittent catheterization
26. Intracranial pressure
27. Computed tomography
28. Process whereby embryonic cells acquire individual characteristics and function

Down

1. Mechanisms leading to an abnormal structure, form, or function
3. A nonrandom occurrence of multiple malformations for which no specific or common etiology has been established
4. Morphogenic defect of an organ or larger region of the body resulting from an abnormal developmental process
5. Perception by nerve endings of traumatic or painful stimuli
7. Overdevelopment of an organ or tissue that results from an increase in the number of cells
9. Cleft lip
13. Endotracheal
15. Arnold-Chiari malformation
16. Central nervous system
22. Neural tube defect
23. Cerebrospinal fluid
25. Magnetic resonance imaging

❖ CHAPTER 12
Health Promotion of the Infant and Family

1. If the infant weighs 7.5 kg at age 6 months, how many kilograms was his/her probable birth weight?
   A. 7.0
   B. 4.0
   C. 3.2
   D. 15.4

2. If the infant's head circumference is 46 cm at 6 months, how many centimeters would you expect his/her head circumference to be at 8 months?
   A. 46.5
   B. 47
   C. 47.5
   D. 49

3. The infant's posterior fontanel usually closes by:
   A. 6 to 8 weeks.
   B. 3 to 6 months.
   C. 12 to 18 months.
   D. 9 to 12 months.

4. Match the neurologic reflex with its expected behavioral response AND the age of its appearance in infancy (one selection from Column 2 and one selection from Column 3).

	Column 2		Column 3
A. labyrinth righting	_____ When infant is suspended in a horizontal prone position and suddenly thrust downward, hand and fingers extend forward as if to protect against falling.	_____	7 to 12 months; persists indefinitely
B. neck righting	_____ When body of an erect infant is tilted, head is returned to upright erect position.	_____	6 months until 24 to 26 months
C. body righting	_____ This is a modification of the neck righting reflex in which turning hips and shoulders to one side causes all other body parts to follow.	_____	2 months; strongest at 10 months
D. otolith righting	_____ When infant is suspended in a horizontal prone position, the head is raised and legs and spine are extended.	_____	6 to 8 months until 12 to 24 months
E. Landau	_____ While infant is supine, head is turned to one side. Shoulder, trunk, and finally pelvis will turn toward that side.	_____	7 to 9 months; persists indefinitely
F. parachute	_____ Infant in prone or supine position is able to raise head.	_____	3 months until 24 to 36 months

5. Which one of the following statements is TRUE about the proportion of the chest at the end of the first year?
   A. The contour of the chest is more like a neonate's than an adult's.
   B. The anteroposterior diameter is larger than the lateral diameter.
   C. The chest is small in relation to the size of the heart.
   D. The chest circumference is about equal to the head circumference.

6. Which one of the following characteristics of vision is developed at the earliest age?
   A. binocularity
   B. stereopsis
   C. corneal reflex
   D. convergence

7. The nurse can expect that an infant will respond to his/her own name by about:
   A. 3 months of age.
   B. 4 months of age.
   C. 6 months of age.
   D. 10 months of age.

8. Which characteristic of the infant's respiratory system predisposes him/her to middle ear infection?
   A. a short, angled eustachian tube
   B. a short, straight eustachian tube
   C. the close proximity of the trachea to the bronchi
   D. the size of the lumen of the eustachian tube

9. Which one of the following hemopoietic changes would be considered abnormal in the first 5 months of life?
   A. low iron levels
   B. physiologic anemia
   C. fetal hemoglobin
   D. low hemoglobin level

10. All of the following digestive processes are deficient in the infant until about 3 months EXCEPT:
    A. amylase.
    B. lipase.
    C. saliva.
    D. trypsin.

11. The _____ is the most immature of all of the gastrointestinal organs throughout infancy.

12. Which one of the following sucking actions is characteristic of the breast-fed infant?
    A. The tongue moves rhythmically forward to the gums and lips and backward.
    B. The infant controls the stream of milk by pushing his/her tongue against the nipple.
    C. The sucking action causes a rapid flow of milk.
    D. The tongue moves from the soft palate to the front of the mouth.

13. Which one of the following is a characteristic of the somatic swallow reflex?
    A. The mandible does not thrust forward.
    B. The tongue is more concave.
    C. It prepares the infant for solids.
    D. It develops before the age of 6 months.

14. After birth, normal levels of immunoglobulin in humans are:
    A. reached by 1 year of age.
    B. reached in early childhood.
    C. transferred from the mother.
    D. reached by 9 months of age.

15. Which one of the following mechanisms decreases the newborn's thermoregulation efficiency?
    A. shivering
    B. limited adipose tissue
    C. dilation of the capillaries
    D. constriction of the capillaries

16. The infant is predisposed to a more rapid loss of total body fluid and dehydration because:
    A. of a high proportion of extracellular fluid.
    B. of a high proportion of intracellular fluid.
    C. total body water is at about 40%.
    D. extracellular fluid is 20% of the total.

17. Complete maturity of the kidney occurs:
    A. at birth.
    B. by 6 months.
    C. by 1 year.
    D. by 24 months.

18. Until the renal structures mature, the range of specific gravity for the infant ranges from 1.__ __ __ to 1.__ __ __.

19. The immaturity of the functioning endocrine system that is normal in the infant will be demonstrated:
    A. in growth patterns.
    B. in thyroid levels.
    C. during times of stress.
    D. in immunoglobulin levels.

20. Fine motor development is evaluated by observing the 10-month-old infant for the:
    A. ability to stack blocks.
    B. pincer grasp.
    C. righting reflexes.
    D. tonic neck reflex.

21. Which one of the following characteristics disappears by about 3 months?
    A. ability to stack blocks
    B. pincer grasp
    C. righting reflexes
    D. tonic neck reflex

22. Which one of the following assessment findings would be considered MOST abnormal?
    A. the infant who displays head lag at 3 months of age
    B. the infant who starts to walk at 18 months
    C. the infant who begins to sit unsupported at 9 months
    D. the infant who begins to roll from front to back at 5 months

23. Which one of the following factors determines the quality of the infant's formulation of trust?
    A. the quality of the interpersonal relationship
    B. the degree of mothering skill
    C. the quantity of the mother's breast milk
    D. the length of suckling time

24. Piaget's theory of cognitive development as it pertains to the infant involves three crucial events:
    A. trust, readjustment, and the regulation of frustration.
    B. separation, object permanence, and mental representation.
    C. imitation, personality development, and temperament.
    D. ordering, comfort, and satisfaction with his/her body.

25. The development of the sexual identity begins:
    A. after the first year.
    B. during the phallic stage.
    C. at birth.
    D. at puberty.

26. Parenting:
    A. is an instinctual ability.
    B. is a learned acquired process.
    C. begins shortly after birth.
    D. shapes the infant's environment positively.

27. Separation anxiety and stranger fear normally begin to appear by:
    A. 4 weeks.
    B. 6 months.
    C. 14 months.
    D. 4 years.

28. Which one of the following play activities would be LEAST appropriate to suggest to the mother for her 3-month-old infant?
    A. playing music and singing along
    B. using rattles
    C. using an infant swing
    D. placing toys a bit out of reach

29. Knowledge of the infant's temperament should NOT be used to help parents to:
    A. see an organized view of the child's behavior.
    B. choose childrearing techniques.
    C. identify a difficult child.
    D. see their child in a better perspective.

30. If a mother is concerned about the fact that her 14-month-old infant is not walking, the nurse would particularly want to evaluate whether the infant:
    A. pulls up on the furniture.
    B. uses a pincer grasp.
    C. transfers objects.
    D. has developed object permanence.

31. If a mother is concerned about "spoiling" her child, the nurse should encourage her to respond to her newborn's crying episodes with:
    A. a delayed response of holding the infant.
    B. a prompt response of holding the infant.
    C. letting the infant cry a little.
    D. maintaining a feeding schedule.

32. Which one of the following could be considered evidence that the child is being spoiled by the parents?
    A. the child who has a difficult temperament and a short attention span
    B. the toddler who has a temper tantrum
    C. the infant who has colic
    D. the child who always cries if he/she doesn't get his/her way

33. Limit setting and discipline should begin in:
    A. middle childhood or adolescence.
    B. infancy with voice tone and eye contact.
    C. early childhood with voice tone and eye contact.
    D. infancy with time out in a chair for misbehavior.

34. In guiding parents who are choosing a day care center, the nurse should stress that state licensure represents a program that maintains:
    A. optimal care.
    B. health features.
    C. minimum requirements.
    D. safety features.

35. A 12-month-old infant would be likely to have:
    A. 2 teeth.
    B. 4 teeth.
    C. 6 teeth.
    D. 12 teeth.

36. Which of the following reasons to put shoes on an infant is CORRECT?
    A. to protect foot from injury
    B. to support foot muscles
    C. to support the ankle
    D. to protect the arch

37. The breast-feeding mother should supplement the breast milk with:
    A. soy-based formula.
    B. milk-based formula.
    C. water.
    D. fluoride.

38. Which one of the following formula feeding patterns would warrant further evaluation for a 1-year-old infant?
    A. four feedings of 5 oz each
    B. five feedings of 8 oz each
    C. three feedings of 6 oz each
    D. four feedings of 6 oz each

39. The primary reason for introducing solids to infants is to:
    A. supply nutrients not found in formula or breast milk.
    B. replace nutrients found in breast milk.
    C. socialize them to the culturally acceptable foods.
    D. promote the disappearance of the extrusion reflex.

40. The risk of botulism can be avoided by sweetening the infant's home-prepared foods with:
    A. honey.
    B. corn syrup.
    C. refined sugar.
    D. none of the above.

41. When introducing new food, the parents should NOT:
    A. decrease the quantity of the infant's milk.
    B. mix food with formula to feed through a nipple.
    C. introduce new foods in small amounts.
    D. offer the new food by itself at first.

42. Match the sleep disturbance with the technique for management.

A. nighttime feeding

B. developmental night crying

C. trained night crying

D. refusal to go to sleep

E. nighttime fear

_____ Check at progressively longer intervals each night.

_____ Keep a night light on.

_____ Reassure parents that this is a temporary phase.

_____ Establish a consistent before-bedtime routine.

_____ Put infant to bed awake.

43. Which one of the following ranges is MOST accurate for the percentage of children under the age of 2 in the United States who are completely vaccinated?
A. 71% to 96%
B. 40% to 58%
C. 11% to 15%
D. 11% to 58%

44. Which one of the following side effects that are MOST likely to occur with an immunization would be considered severe?
A. febrile episode
B. malaise
C. encephalitis
D. behavioral changes

45. The nurse should withhold immunization with the oral polio vaccine if which one of the following situations exists?
A. The child had a temperature of 104° after the last immunization.
B. The child has a cold with a temperature of 100°.
C. The child has had a kidney transplant.
D. The child had a seizure the day after the last immunization.

46. Which one of the following techniques has been demonstrated by research to minimize local reactions when administering immunizations to infants?
A. Select a 1-inch needle to deposit the vaccine deep in the muscle mass.
B. Use an air bubble to clear the needle after the injection.
C. Change the needle on the syringe after drawing up the vaccine.
D. Apply a topical anesthetic to the site for a minimum of one hour.

47. To prevent aspiration in the infant, the nurse should avoid using:
A. baby powder made from cornstarch.
B. pacifiers made from a padded nipple.
C. syringes to dispense oral medication.
D. pacifiers with one-piece construction.

48. Which one of the following hazards causes the majority of deaths in young children?
A. plastic garment bags
B. ill-fitting crib slats
C. latex balloons
D. ill-fitting crib mattresses

49. Which one of the following situations involving cords would be considered LEAST hazardous?
A. a bib that is not removed at bedtime
B. a pacifier that is hung around the infant's neck with a 10-inch string
C. a play telephone with a 10-inch cord
D. a toy tied to the playpen with a 15-inch ribbon

50. The BEST place in the car for the infant car restraint is in the:
    A. middle of the back seat, facing back.
    B. middle of the back seat, facing front.
    C. passenger seat with an air bag, facing front.
    D. passenger seat with an air bag, facing back.

51. To prevent falls, the parents should take all of the following precautions EXCEPT:
    A. never leave the child on a changing table unattended.
    B. keep necessary articles within easy reach.
    C. change the infant's diaper on the floor.
    D. use a walker to strengthen the walking muscles.

52. One way to distract an infant while changing his/her diaper that should NOT be recommended is to:
    A. give the infant the bottle of talc baby powder to hold.
    B. sing and play with the infant.
    C. play the same game each time.
    D. None of the above are recommended.

❖ Critical Thinking ❖
Case Study

Jennifer Klein, a 6-month-old infant, is admitted to the Pediatric Unit with bronchiolitis. Both of her parents work and the baby attends day care. Jennifer is the first child, and the parents seem anxious about the admission as well as her care at home and her normal development. It is clear that the parents need information about general health promotion for their infant.

53. Which areas should be assessed to determine the status of the parents' current health promotion practices? (Check all that apply.)

_____ respiratory status (lung sounds)

_____ nutrition

_____ fever patterns

_____ sleep and activity

_____ number and condition of teeth

_____ fluid and hydration status

_____ condition of the mucous membranes of the mouth

_____ immunization status

_____ safety precautions used in the home

54. Which one of the following nursing diagnoses would be used MOST often for health promotion related to development in an infant Jennifer's age?
   A. activity intolerance
   B. ineffective thermoregulation
   C. high risk for injury
   D. altered parenting

55. Which one of the following strategies is used MOST often to help new parents like Jennifer's adjust to the parenting role?
   A. parenting classes
   B. anticipatory guidance
   C. first aid courses
   D. cardiopulmonary resuscitation courses

56. By the time Jennifer is ready for discharge, the nurse evaluates that her parents have achieved improved parenting skills. Which one of the following methods would BEST measure the plan's success?
   A. Jennifer is afebrile.
   B. Reports from the other staff are positive.
   C. Verbalizations from the parents indicate that they understand.
   D. A home visit demonstrates that positive changes have occurred.

❖ Crossword Puzzle ❖

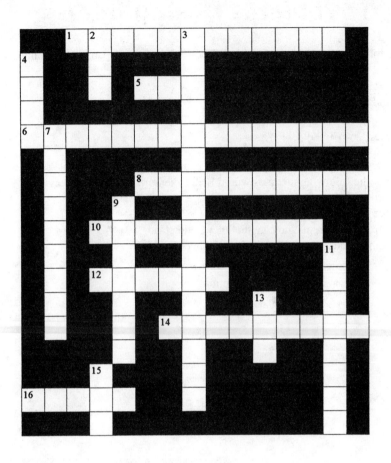

Across

1. Play that is centered on own activities (2 words)
5. Infant Temperament Questionnaire
6. Temporary immunity by transfusing plasma proteins artificially or naturally from one who has been actively immunized against an antigen (2 words)
8. Depth perception
10. Self-love
12. Pattern of action and/or thought
14. Antibody formed in response to a toxin
16. National Childhood Vaccine Injury Act

Down

2. Oral polio virus
3. Immunity from exposure to the invading host (2 words)
4. Advisory Committee on Immunization Practices
7. Reduce the virulence of a pathogenic microorganism
9. Any type of active immunization agent
11. A protein that is formed in response to exposure to a specific antigen
13. Diphtheria, tetanus, pertussis
15. Tetanus immune globulin

❖ CHAPTER 13
Health Problems During Infancy

1. In the United States, which of the following populations is at highest risk for developing a vitamin D deficiency?
   A. lower socioeconomic groups
   B. those that use raw cow's milk
   C. children with measles
   D. children with rheumatoid arthritis

2. The greatest concern with minerals is:
   A. deficiency.
   B. excess causing toxicity.
   C. nervous system disturbances from excess.
   D. hemochromatosis.

3. Match the type of vegetarianism with its description.

   A. lacto-ovovegetarians   _____ This group eliminates any food of animal origin, including milk and
                                            eggs.

   B. lactovegetarians
                                    _____ This group is most restrictive of all. Brown rice is the mainstay of
   C. pure vegetarians (vegans)   the diet.

   D. Zen macrobiotics   _____ This group excludes meat from their diet but eats milk, eggs, and
                                            sometimes fish.

                                    _____ This group excludes meat and eggs but drinks milk.

4. What nutrient should the nutritional assessment evaluate for any family who is vegetarian? _____

5. Which one of the following sources applies to children and should be used to convey nutrition information to the public?
   A. Recommended Dietary Allowances (RDAs)
   B. the basic four food groups
   C. Food Guide Pyramid
   D. Dietary Guidelines for Americans

6. Which of the following combinations of foods would ensure the most complete protein for a strictly vegetarian family if eaten together at the same meal?
   A. milk and chicken
   B. sunflower seeds and rice
   C. rice and red beans
   D. eggs and cheese

7. In the United States, protein and energy malnutrition (PEM) occurs where:
   A. the food supply is inadequate.
   B. the food supply may be adequate.
   C. the adults eat first, leaving insufficient food.
   D. the diet consists mainly of starch grains.

8. Kwashiorkor results in populations where:
   A. the food supply is inadequate.
   B. the food supply is adequate for protein.
   C. the adults eat first, leaving insufficient food.
   D. the diet consists mainly of starch grains.

9. Nutritional marasmus usually results in populations where:
   A. the food supply is inadequate.
   B. the food supply is adequate for protein.
   C. the adults eat first, leaving insufficient food.
   D. the diet consists mainly of starch grains.

10. Which one of the following therapeutic management treatments would be considered INAPPROPRIATE for PEM, kwashiorkor, or marasmus?
    A. Provide high-protein, high-carbohydrate diet.
    B. Replace fluids and electrolytes.
    C. Provide a high-fiber, high-fat diet.
    D. Provide a structured play program.

11. Obesity in adults has been shown to be linked to:
    A. adolescent obesity.
    B. infant obesity.
    C. breast-feeding.
    D. bottle-feeding.

12. The primary goal in regard to obesity in infants is:
    A. safe weight loss.
    B. prevention.
    C. decrease the fat content in the milk.
    D. decrease the total quantity of food.

13. Which one of the following foods is NOT generally considered allergenic?
    A. orange juice
    B. eggs
    C. bread
    D. rice

14. Which one of the following clinical manifestations may indicate that an infant has an allergy to cow's milk?
    A. sleeplessness
    B. colic
    C. vomiting and diarrhea
    D. all of the above

15. Which one of the following diagnostic strategies is the MOST definitive for identifying a milk allergy?
    A. stool analysis for blood
    B. serum IgE levels
    C. a challenge of milk after elimination
    D. skin testing

16. Treatment of cow's milk allergy in infants involves changing the formula to:
    A. soy-based formula.
    B. goat's milk.
    C. casein/whey hydrolysate milk.
    D. breast milk.

17. Congenital lactose intolerance refers to:
    A. a rare form of lactose intolerance.
    B. a form of lactose intolerance associated with giardiasis.
    C. an intolerance manifested later in life.
    D. all of the above.

18. Match the common breast-feeding problem with the appropriate strategy.

    A. engorgement   _____   may need to use oxytocin nasal spray

    B. painful nipples   _____   prevent this problem with frequent feedings

    C. let-down reflex   _____   have infant nurse on the unaffected side first

    D. inadequate milk supply   _____   may need antibiotics to treat this problem

    E. plugged ducts   _____   avoid use of supplemental feedings

    F. mastitis   _____   position infant's chin toward affected area

19. If a sensitivity to cow's milk is suspected as the cause of an infant's colic, the parents should:
    A. try substituting casein hydrolysate formula.
    B. try substituting soy formula.
    C. be reassured that the symptoms will disappear spontaneously at about 3 months of age.
    D. be assessed for improper feeding techniques.

20. Which of the following phrases BEST defines *rumination*?
    A. It is the involuntary return of undigested food from the stomach, usually accompanied by burping.
    B. It is the dribbling of unswallowed formula from the infant's mouth immediately after a feeding.
    C. It is the active, voluntary return of swallowed food into the mouth.
    D. It is the same as vomiting.

21. Which one of the following strategies for management of colic in a 6-month-old infant is CONTRAINDICATED?
    A. Use soy formula.
    B. dicyclomine hydrochloride
    C. hydroxyzine hydrochloride
    D. Avoid smoking.

22. If failure to thrive has been a long-standing problem, the infant will have evidence of:
    A. weight and height depression.
    B. weight depression only.
    C. height depression only.
    D. emotional deprivation.

23. Which one of the following characteristics in an infant with failure to thrive would be MOST significant?
    A. difficult feeding pattern with vomiting and aversion behavior
    B. crying, excessive irritability, and sleep pattern disturbances
    C. lack of congruence between the child's temperament and that of the parents
    D. irregularity in activities of daily living and difficult temperament pattern

24. Which one of the following strategies might be recommended for an infant with failure to thrive to increase the caloric intake?
    A. Utilize developmental stimulation by a specialist during feedings.
    B. Avoid solids until after the bottle is well accepted.
    C. Be persistent through 10 to 15 minutes of food refusal.
    D. Vary the schedule for routine activities on a daily basis.

25. The incidence of diaper dermatitis is generally reported as greater in bottle-fed infants than in breast-fed infants, because in breast-fed infants there is a lower:
    A. ammonia content of the urine.
    B. pH content of the feces.
    C. microbial content of the feces.
    D. number of stools per day.

26. Which one of the following strategies should the nurse recommend to the parents of an infant with diaper dermatitis?
    A. Apply fluorinated hydrocortisone sparingly.
    B. Avoid cornstarch because it promotes yeast growth.
    C. Use a hand-held dryer on the open lesions.
    D. Use diapers with super-absorbent gelling material.

27. Which one of the following strategies for the care of atopic dermatitis is controversial?
    A. Use the wet method of skin care.
    B. Use the dry method of skin care.
    C. Limit the infant's exposure to allergens.
    D. Avoid exposure of the infant to skin irritants.

28. Identify the following statements as either TRUE or FALSE.

    _____ The incidence of sudden infant death syndrome (SIDS) is associated with diphtheria, tetanus, and pertussis vaccines.

    _____ Maternal smoking during and after pregnancy has been implicated as a contributor to SIDS.

    _____ Parents should be advised to position an infant on his/her abdomen to prevent SIDS.

    _____ The nurse should encourage the parents to sleep in the same bed as the infant being monitored for apnea of infancy in order to detect subtle clinical changes.

    _____ The psychogenic theory of autism which is unsupported by current findings depicts the parents of the autistic child as detached individuals.

❖ Critical Thinking ❖
Case Study

Six-month-old Jason Fitch has come to the office today for his routine immunizations. His mother says she thinks everything is just fine, except that Jason seems to have a lot of food intolerances.

The nurse continues the assessment and finds that Jason is eating many of the food items the rest of the family eats, including milk products in very small amounts. There is no particular pattern to the way the new foods are being introduced.

Jason exhibits a variety of symptoms related to skin irritations. He is developing rashes around his mouth and rectum and elsewhere on his body when he eats certain foods.

29. Based on the prevalence of common health problems of infancy, what areas should the nurse include in Jason's initial assessment?
    A. nutrition
    B. temperament
    C. sleep patterns
    D. all of the above

30. Based on the data from the assessment interview, which one of the following goals would be BEST for the nurse to establish?
    A. to prevent outbreaks of food allergy
    B. to prevent death from anaphylaxis
    C. to prevent genetic transmission
    D. all of the above

31. Which one of the following recommendations would be MOST appropriate for Jason's mother?
    A. Reconsider breast-feeding.
    B. Eliminate cow's milk.
    C. Introduce only one new food at each five-day interval.
    D. Eliminate solids until 9 months of age.

32. At an earlier visit, the nurse had determined that there was altered parenting related to lack of knowledge in Jason's family. Which one of the following outcome criteria would help the nurse evaluate the mother's ability to provide a constructive environment for Jason in regard to this diagnosis of altered parenting? Jason's mother is able to:
    A. identify eating patterns that contribute to symptoms.
    B. share feelings regarding her parenting skills.
    C. practice appropriate precautions to prevent infection.
    D. identify the rationale for prevention of the skin rashes.

❖ Crossword Puzzle ❖

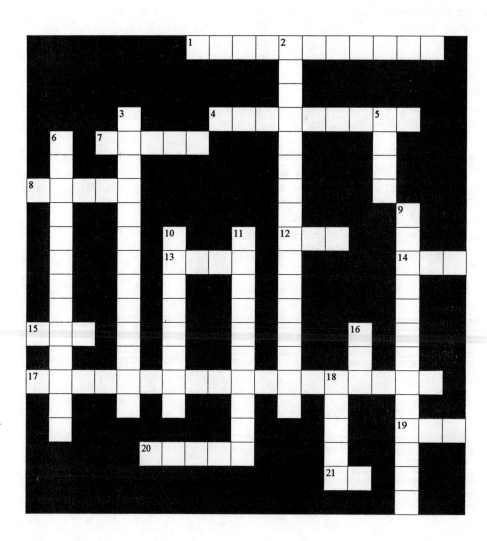

Across

1. Protein deficiency with low or adequate energy sources
4. Proteins that are capable of inducing IgE antibody formation when ingested, inhaled, or injected
7. Individual who excludes all animal products from the diet
8. Nursing Child Assessment Feeding Scale
12. Apnea of infancy
13. Apparent life-threatening event
14. Cardiopulmonary resuscitation
15. Protein-energy malnutrition
17. A, D, E, and K (3 words)
19. Recommended dietary allowance
20. Allergy with tendency to be inherited
21. Atopic dermatitis

Down

2. Excessive intake of a vitamin that causes adverse clinical effects
3. Initial exposure to an allergen, resulting in an immune response
5. Nonorganic failure to thrive
6. Minerals for which daily requirements are greater than 100 mg
9. Trace elements
10. State of semistarvation from inadequate protein and energy
11. Inadequate intake of a nutrient that causes adverse clinical effects
16. Absorbent gelling material
18. Respiratory pause of more than 20 seconds

❖ CHAPTER 14
Health Promotion of the Toddler and Family

1. If the chest circumference of a toddler is 50 cm, how many cm would you expect the head circumference to be?
   A. 25
   B. 35
   C. 50
   D. 60

2. Which one of the following factors is MOST important in predisposing toddlers to frequent infections?
   A. There is a short straight internal ear canal and large lymph tissue.
   B. Pulse and respiratory rate are slower and blood pressure increases.
   C. Respirations are abdominal.
   D. The defense mechanisms are less efficient than during infancy.

3. One of the MOST important digestive system changes that is completed during the toddler period is the:
   A. increased acidity of the gastric contents.
   B. voluntary control of the sphincters.
   C. protective function of the gastric contents.
   D. increased capacity of the stomach.

4. Which one of the following statements is MOST characteristic of the motor skills of a 24-month-old?
   A. Motor skills are fully developed but occur in isolation from the environment.
   B. The toddler walks alone but falls easily.
   C. The toddler's activities begin to produce purposeful results.
   D. The toddler is able to grasp small objects but cannot release them at will.

5. Using Erikson's theory as a foundation, the primary developmental task of the toddler period is to:
   A. satisfy the need for basic trust.
   B. achieve a sense of accomplishment.
   C. learn to give up dependence for independence.
   D. acquire language or mental symbolism.

6. Piaget's theory of cognitive development depicts the toddler as a child who:
   A. continuously explores the same object each time it appears in a new place.
   B. is able to transfer information from one situation to another.
   C. has a persistent negative response to any request.
   D. has a rudimentary beginning of a superego.

7. According to Kohlberg, the BEST way to discipline children is to:
   A. use a punishment and obedience orientation.
   B. withhold privileges.
   C. use power to control behavior.
   D. give explanations and help the child to change.

8. By the age of 2, the toddler generally:
   A. has clear body boundaries.
   B. participates willingly in most procedures.
   C. recognizes sexual differences.
   D. is unable to learn correct terms for body parts.

9. Which of the following skills is NOT necessary for the toddler to acquire before separation and individuation can be achieved?
   A. object permanence
   B. lack of anxiety during separations from parents
   C. delayed gratification
   D. ability to tolerate a moderate amount of frustration

10. The usual number of words acquired by the age of 2 years is about:
   A. 50.
   B. 100.
   C. 300.
   D. 500.

11. The 2-year-old child living in a bilingual environment will generally have:
   A. advanced speaking ability without adequate comprehension.
   B. advanced speaking ability with advanced comprehension.
   C. delayed speaking ability with adequate comprehension.
   D. delayed speaking ability without adequate comprehension.

12. Which one of the following types of play decreases in frequency as the child moves through the toddler period?
   A. solitary play
   B. imitative play
   C. tactile play
   D. parallel play

13. Which one of the following statements is FALSE in regard to toilet training?
   A. Bowel training is usually accomplished after bladder training.
   B. Nighttime bladder training is usually accomplished after bowel training.
   C. The toddler who is impatient with soiled diapers is demonstrating readiness for toilet training.
   D. Fewer wet diapers signals that the toddler is physically ready for toilet training.

14. Which one of the following strategies is appropriate for parents to use to prepare a toddler for the birth of a sibling?
   A. Explain the upcoming birth as early in the pregnancy as possible.
   B. Move the toddler to his/her own new room.
   C. Provide a doll for the toddler to imitate parenting.
   D. Tell the toddler that a new playmate will come home soon.

15. The BEST approach for extinguishing a toddler's attention-seeking behavior of a tantrum with head banging is to:
   A. ignore the behavior.
   B. provide time out.
   C. offer a toy to calm the child.
   D. protect the child from injury.

16. Which one of the following techniques is BEST to deal with the negativism of the toddler?
   A. Quietly and calmly ask the child to comply.
   B. Provide few or no choices for the child.
   C. Challenge the child with a game.
   D. Remain serious and intent.

17. Which of the following statements about stress in toddlers is TRUE?
   A. Toddlers are rarely exposed to stress or the results of stress.
   B. Any stress is destructive because toddlers have a limited ability to cope.
   C. Most children are exposed to a stress-free environment.
   D. Small amounts of stress help toddlers develop effective coping skills.

18. Regression in toddlers occurs when there is:
    A. stress.
    B. a threat to their autonomy.
    C. a need to revert to dependency.
    D. all of the above.

19. Which of the following statements is TRUE in regard to nutritional changes from the infant to the toddler years?
    A. Caloric requirements increase from 102 kcal/kg to 108 kcal/kg.
    B. Caloric requirements decrease from 108 kcal/kg to 102 kcal/kg.
    C. Protein requirements decrease from 2.2 kcal/kg to 1.5 kcal/kg.
    D. Protein requirements increase from 1.2 kcal/kg to 2.2 kcal/kg.

20. Reduced fluid requirement in toddlers represents a decrease in total body fluid with:
    A. an increase in intracellular fluid.
    B. an increase in extracellular fluid.
    C. a decrease in intracellular fluid.
    D. a decrease in extracellular fluid.

21. Which one of the following nutritional requirements increases during the toddler years?
    A. calories
    B. proteins
    C. minerals
    D. fluids

22. Physiologic anorexia in toddlers is characterized by:
    A. strong taste preferences.
    B. extreme changes in appetite from day to day.
    C. heightened awareness of social aspects of meals.
    D. all of the above.

23. Healthy ways of serving food to toddlers include:
    A. requiring a pattern of sitting at a table for meals.
    B. permitting nutritious nibbling.
    C. discouraging between-meal snacking.
    D. all of the above.

24. Developmentally, most children at 12 months:
    A. use a spoon adeptly.
    B. relinquish the bottle voluntarily.
    C. eat the same food as the rest of the family.
    D. reject all solid food in preference for the bottle.

25. The BEST approach to use for the toddler who prefers the bottle to all solid food is to:
    A. require the toddler to eat something.
    B. dilute the milk with water.
    C. withhold all food and water until the child takes solids.
    D. puree the solids and feed them through the bottle.

26. For a toddler with sleep problems, the nurse should suggest:
    A. using a transitional object.
    B. varying the bedtime ritual.
    C. restricting stimulating activities.
    D. all of the above.

27. Which one of the following strategies is INAPPROPRIATE for the parent to use to help the toddler adjust to the initial dental visit?
    A. Explain to the child that a checkup won't hurt.
    B. Have the child observe his/her brother's examination.
    C. Have the child perform a checkup on a doll.
    D. Ask the dentist to reserve a thorough examination for another visit.

28. The MOST effective way to clean a toddler's teeth is:
    A. for the child to brush regularly with a toothpaste of his/her choice.
    B. for the parent to stabilize the chin with one hand and brush with the other.
    C. for the parent to brush the mandibular occlusive surfaces, leaving the rest for the child.
    D. for the parent to brush the front labial surface, leaving the rest for the child.

29. Flossing is necessary:
    A. only after the permanent teeth erupt.
    B. to prevent fluorosis.
    C. for the toddler to learn.
    D. even if teeth are widely spaced.

30. Adequate fluoride ingestion:
    A. prevents gingivitis.
    B. prevents fluorosis.
    C. alters the anatomy of the tooth.
    D. reduces the amount of plaque.

31. Recommendations for toddlers to meet fluoride requirements include all of the following EXCEPT:
    A. supervise the use of toothpaste.
    B. supervise the use of fluoride rinse.
    C. store fluoride products out of reach.
    D. administer fluoride supplements if water fluoride content is low.

32. One example of a snack that may actually damage the teeth is:
    A. aged cheese.
    B. celery sticks.
    C. sugarless gum.
    D. a handful of raisins.

33. Which of the following practices contributes to nursing bottle caries?
    A. using a pacifier
    B. feeding the last bottle before bedtime
    C. long, frequent nocturnal breast-feeding
    D. all of the above

34. Match the major developmental achievement of the young child with the safety precaution that could be used to prevent injury.

A. depth perception undefined	_____	Do not allow child to play near curb or parked cars.
B. able to open most containers	_____	Choose large toys without sharp edges.
C. unaware of most dangers	_____	Supervise closely at all times.
D. walks, runs, and moves quickly	_____	Do not allow lollipop or similar objects when walking or running.
E. puts things in mouth	_____	Remove unsecured or scatter rugs.
F. easily distracted	_____	Know the phone number of poison control center.

35. _____ _____ injuries cause more accidental deaths in all pediatric age groups.

36. Children should use convertible car restraints until:
    A. they weigh 40 pounds.
    B. they reach 40 inches in height.
    C. the midpoint of the head is higher than the vehicle seat back.
    D. all of the above

37. One of the BEST ways to prevent drowning in toddlers is for parents to:
    A. learn cardiopulmonary resuscitation (CPR).
    B. supervise children whenever they are near any source of water.
    C. enroll the toddler in a swimming program.
    D. all of the above

38. The MOST common cause of burns in the toddler age group is the:
    A. flame burn from playing with matches.
    B. scald burn from high-temperature tap water or hot liquids.
    C. hot object burn from cigarettes or irons.
    D. electric burn from electrical outlets.

39. The MOST fatal type of burn in the toddler age group is:
    A. flame burn from playing with matches.
    B. scald burn from high-temperature tap water or hot liquids.
    C. hot object burn from cigarettes or irons.
    D. electric burn from electrical outlets.

40. Poisonings in toddlers can be BEST prevented by:
    A. consistently using safety caps.
    B. storing poisonous substances in a locked cabinet.
    C. keeping ipecac syrup in the home.
    D. storing poisonous substances out of reach.

41. The parents should consider moving the toddler from the crib to a bed after the toddler:
    A. reaches the age of 2 years.
    B. will stay in the bed all night.
    C. reaches a height of 35 inches.
    D. is able to sleep through the night.

42. Give an example of an item that could cause aspiration or suffocation for each category of items hazardous to the toddler (e.g., Foods: hard candy).

    Foods: _____

    Play objects: _____

    Common household objects: _____

    Electrical items: _____

❖ Critical Thinking ❖
Case Study

Tasha Jackson is a 12-month-old infant who is visiting the clinic for her well baby checkup. Tasha's mother, Dora, is expecting her second child in three months. Dora works full-time and will be home for six weeks with the new baby. Tasha has been in day care since she was a baby. Mr. Jackson also works full-time during the day.

43. List at least four areas that should by assessed by the nurse to obtain the information necessary to adequately give anticipatory guidance for a toddler at Tasha's age.

   _____

   _____

   _____

   _____

44. Which one of the following nursing interventions would be MOST appropriate to implement?
    A. Allow Ms. Jackson to express her feelings.
    B. Give Ms. Jackson advice about day care.
    C. Give Ms. Jackson advice about sibling rivalry.
    D. all of the above

45. Dora Jackson shares with the nurse that she is concerned about her day care and is thinking about keeping Tasha at home for the six weeks after the baby is born. Which intervention has the highest priority in this situation?
    A. Stress the importance of preparing Tasha for the new sibling.
    B. Recommend that Ms. Jackson begin making plans to keep Tasha at home for the six weeks.
    C. Recommend that any change in day care should take place well before the new baby's arrival.
    D. Explore Ms. Jackson's concerns about her day care arrangements.

46. Which evaluation method would BEST delineate whether Ms. Jackson's concerns were warranted?
    A. a home visit after the baby is born
    B. a visit to the day care center
    C. a return demonstration of baby care
    D. verbalization from Ms. Jackson that she is comfortable with her postpartum arrangements

❖ Crossword Puzzle ❖

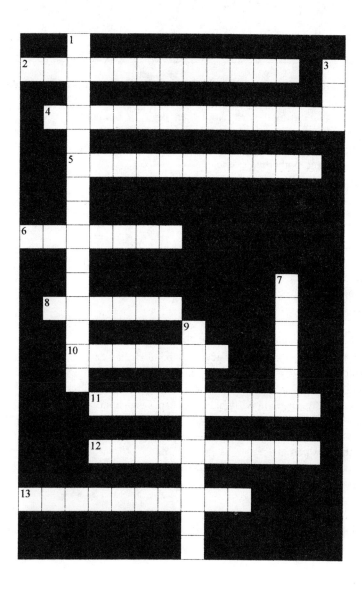

Across

2. Playing alongside but not with other children (2 words)
4. Sudden, explosive outbursts of anger (2 words)
5. Inability to take another's viewpoint
6. Ascribing lifelike qualities to inanimate objects
8. Soft bacterial deposits that form on the teeth
10. Child ages 12 to 36 months
11. Persistent negative response to requests
12. Ability to cognitively manipulate objects
13. Retreat from persistent pattern of functioning to past levels of behavior

Down

1. Unable to undo mentally an action that is initiated physically
3. Absorbent gelling material
7. Decayed areas on teeth
9. Tendency to focus on one aspect of object or event

❖ CHAPTER 15
Health Promotion of the Preschooler and Family

1. The approximate age range for the preschool period begins at age _____ years and ends at age _____ years.

2. The average annual weight gain during the preschool years is _____ pounds.

3. Which one the following statements about the preschooler's physical proportions is TRUE?
   A. Preschoolers have a squat and potbellied frame.
   B. Preschoolers have a slender but sturdy frame.
   C. The muscle and bones of the preschooler have matured.
   D. Sexual characteristics can be differentiated in the preschooler.

4. Uninhibited scribbling and drawing can help to develop:
   A. symbolic language.
   B. fine muscle skills.
   C. eye-hand coordination.
   D. all of the above.

5. To prevent injuries in preschoolers, parents should be able to:
   A. supervise them constantly.
   B. keep them within sight.
   C. enforce limits verbally.
   D. all of the above

6. The resolution of the Oedipus/Electra complex occurs when the child:
   A. identifies with the same-sex parent.
   B. realizes that the same-sex parent is more powerful.
   C. wishes that the same-sex parent were dead.
   D. notices physical sexual differences.

7. Because of the preschooler's egocentric thought, the BEST approach for effective communication is through:
   A. speech.
   B. play.
   C. drawing.
   D. actions.

8. Magical thinking according to Piaget is the belief that:
   A. events have cause and effect.
   B. God is like an imaginary friend.
   C. thoughts are all-powerful.
   D. if the skin is broken, their insides will come out.

9. The moral and spiritual development of the preschooler is characterized by:
   A. concern for why something is wrong.
   B. actions that are directed toward satisfying the needs of others.
   C. thoughts of loyalty and gratitude.
   D. a very concrete sense of justice.

10. The preschooler's body image has developed to include:
    A. a well-defined body boundary.
    B. knowledge about his/her internal anatomy.
    C. fear of intrusive experiences.
    D. anxiety and fear of separation.

11. Sex typing involves the process by which the preschooler:
    A. forms a strong attachment to the same-sex parent.
    B. identifies with the opposite-sex parent.
    C. develops sexual orientation.
    D. all of the above

12. Which one of the following statements about social development of the preschooler is FALSE?
    A. Imaginary playmates are a normal part of the preschooler's play.
    B. Preschoolers have overcome much of their anxiety regarding strangers.
    C. Preschoolers use telegraphic speech between the ages of 3 and 4 years.
    D. Preschoolers particularly enjoy parallel play.

13. In regard to the development of temperament in the preschool years:
    A. temperamental characteristics change considerably during the preschool years.
    B. the effect of temperament on adjustment in a group becomes important during the preschool years.
    C. children need to be treated the same regardless of differences in temperament.
    D. there really is no tool that will adequately identify temperamental characteristics during the preschool years.

14. Recently concern has focused on day care programs that:
    A. stress formal academics.
    B. prepare the child for kindergarten.
    C. provide a structured day.
    D. all of the above

15. Which one of the following descriptions explains the difference between readiness testing and developmental screening?
    A. Developmental screening is used to evaluate counting and writing skills; readiness testing addresses cognitive and physical milestones.
    B. Developmental screening focuses on the skills acquired; readiness testing stresses the potential to learn.
    C. Developmental screening is used to prepare the child for preschool; readiness testing addresses counting and writing skills.
    D. Developmental screening focuses on the potential to learn; readiness testing stresses the skills acquired.

16. The BEST way for parents to respond to questions about sexuality is to give the child:
    A. an honest answer and find out what the child thinks.
    B. one or two sentences that answer the specific question only.
    C. an honest, short, and to-the-point answer.
    D. an honest answer and a little less information than the child expects.

17. Which one of the following characteristics is NOT typically seen in a gifted child?
    A. constant questioning
    B. play with imaginary friend
    C. extremely mature social skills
    D. temperamental

18. Which one of the following factors influences aggressive behavior?
    A. frustration
    B. modeling
    C. gender
    D. all of the above

19. Which one of the following dysfunctional speech patterns is a normal characteristic of the language development of a preschool-age child?

    A. lisp

    B. stammering

    C. nystagmus

    D. echolalia

20. Which one of the following sources of stress in the preschool-age child is typical of a 3-year-old?

    A. insecurity

    B. masturbation

    C. jealousy

    D. sexuality

21. Which one of the following approaches is recommended to help prevent stress in children?

    A. Allow time for rest.

    B. Prepare the child for changes.

    C. Monitor the amount of stress.

    D. all of the above

22. Which one of the following examples would BEST help a preschool child dispel his/her fear of the water when learning to swim?

    A. Fear of the water is a healthy fear. It should not be dispelled.

    B. Allow the child to sit by the water with other children, play with water toys, and get splashed lightly with the water.

    C. Reassure the child as he/she is brought slowly into the water with an adult who knows how to swim.

    D. Throw the child in the water and have an adult keep the child's head above water.

23. Preschool children with reported sleep problems sleep (circle one) MORE or LESS than children without sleep difficulties.

24. Identify the following statements as either TRUE or FALSE.

    _____ Sleep terrors can be described as a partial arousal from a very deep non-dreaming sleep.

    _____ Nightmares usually occur in the second half of the night.

    _____ With sleep terrors, crying and fright persist even after the child is awake.

    _____ With nightmares, the child is not very aware of another's presence.

25. When educating the preschool child about injury prevention, the parents should:

    A. set a good example.

    B. help children establish good habits.

    C. be aware that pedestrian/motor vehicle injuries increase in this age group.

    D. all of the above

❖ Critical Thinking ❖
Case Study

Sheila Roth arrives at the office for a routine preschool physical. Her son Jacob, who is not quite 3 years old, will attend the preschool program for 3-year-olds at a local private school this year. He has attended a home day care program since he was a baby, while his mother tends to her own interior decorating business.

The day care is run by an older woman who treats the twelve children in her program as if they were family. The helper at the day care is also very loving. The program is very structured in regard to schedule and usual routines.

Ms. Roth tells the nurse that she is really looking forward to Jacob's new environment. His teacher is very creative and approaches the classroom from the perspective of the child's development. There will be a lot of choices for activities during the day.

26. Based on the information above, which one of the following is the BEST analysis of the data presented?
    A. Jacob needs some preparation for this new preschool experience.
    B. Jacob will have less trouble adjusting than a child who has never attended day care.
    C. Jacob is too young for such a drastic change.
    D. Jacob needs the individual attention he is getting at the day care.

27. Which one of the following expected outcomes would be MOST reasonable to establish?
    A. The nurse will help Ms. Roth assess Jacob's readiness for preschool.
    B. Jacob will attend preschool without any behavioral indications of stress.
    C. Ms. Roth will verbalize at least five strategies that can be used to help prepare Jacob for his preschool experience.
    D. Jacob will demonstrate behavior that indicates he is adjusting to his preschool experience.

28. Which one of the following interventions would be INAPPROPRIATE for the nurse to suggest?
    A. Introduce Jacob to the teacher.
    B. Leave quickly the first day.
    C. Talk about the new school as exciting.
    D. Be confident the first day.

29. Which one of the following of Jacob's characteristics would indicate that he is ready for preschool?
    A. social maturity
    B. good attention span
    C. academically ready
    D. all of the above

❖ Crossword Puzzle ❖

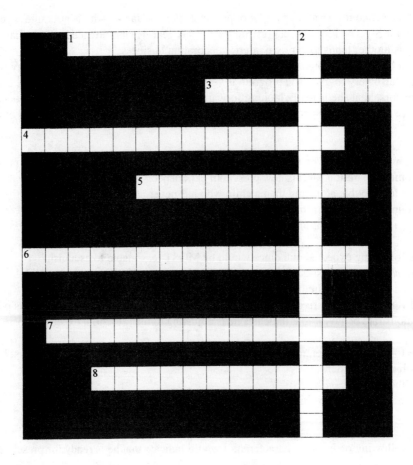

Across

1. Period in which children's designs become recognizable as familiar objects (2 words)
3. Imitating behavior of significant others
4. Period in which children put spontaneous scribblings on paper in a specific pattern (2 words)
5. Period in which children draw outline forms (2 words)
6. Belief that thoughts are powerful and cause events (2 words)
7. Group play of similar or identical activities but without rigid rules (2 words)
8. Child ages 3 to 5 years

Down

2. Children's sentences that contain 3 to 4 essential words (2 words)

❖ CHAPTER 16
Health Problems of Early Childhood

1. Match the communicable disease term with its definition.

A. communicable disease

_____ provides subsistence or lodging to infectious agent

B. epidemic

_____ harbors infectious agent without apparent disease

C. endemic

_____ person or animal that has been in association with source that could provide the infected agent

D. infectious agent

_____ illness caused by specific infectious agent through some transmission of agent

E. reservoir

F. host

_____ disease occurring regularly within a geographic location

G. carrier

_____ disease occurring in greater than expected numbers within a community

H. contact

I. direct

_____ environment in which infectious agent lives and multiplies

J. vehicle

_____ organism that is capable of producing infection

K. incubation period

_____ contact and immediate transfer of infectious agent by kissing

L. period of communicability

_____ an object serving as intermediate means for transportation of infectious agent

_____ time period when infection may be directly or indirectly transported

_____ time from exposure to appearance of symptoms

2. Match the communicable disease with the statement.

A. varicella

_____ Rash appears in three stages. Stage I is erythema on face, chiefly on cheeks.

B. diphtheria

_____ begins as macule rash, rapidly progresses to papule rash, then vesicles, and then breaks and forms crusts

C. fifth disease

_____ Tonsillar pharyngeal areas are covered with white or gray membrane. Complications include myocarditis and neuritis.

D. roseola

E. rubeola

_____ Rash is rose-pink macules or maculopapules appearing first on trunk, then neck, face, and extremities. It is a nonpruritic rash.

F. mumps

_____ Cough occurs at night, and inspirations sound like crowing.

G. pertussis

_____ earache that is aggravated by chewing

H. rubella

_____ Rash appears three to four days after onset and maculopapular eruption on face with gradual spread downward. Koplik spots present before rash.

I. scarlet fever

J. poliomyelitis

_____ Discrete pinkish red maculopapular rash appears on face and then downward to neck, arms, trunk, and legs. Greatest danger is teratogenic effect on fetus.

_____ can have permanent paralysis

_____ Tonsils are enlarged, edematous, reddened, and covered with patches of exudate. Rash is absent on face. Desquamation occurs.

3. Assessment of which of the following is NOT helpful in identifying potentially communicable diseases?
   A. recent travel to foreign country
   B. immunization history
   C. past medical history
   D. family history

4. Primary prevention of communicable disease is BEST accomplished by:
   A. immunization.
   B. control of the disease spread.
   C. adequate water supply.
   D. implementing good handwashing among hospital personnel.

5. Certain groups of children are at risk for serious complications from communicable diseases. These children include which of the following groups?
   A. children with an immunodeficiency or immunologic disorder
   B. children receiving steroid therapy
   C. children with leukemia
   D. all of the above

6. What antiviral agent is used to treat varicella infections in children at increased risk for complications associated with varicella?
   A. varicella-zoster immune globulin
   B. acyclovir
   C. salicylates
   D. all of the above

7. A major responsibility of the school nurse working with children at high risk for communicable diseases is to

_____.

8. The American Academy of Pediatrics has recommended vitamin A supplements for certain pediatric patients with measles. Correct dosage of vitamin A and instruction to parents of these children include:
   1. single oral dose of 200,000 IU in children 1 year old.
   2. single oral dose of 100,000 IU in children 6 to 12 months old.
   3. dosage may be associated with vomiting and headache for a few hours.
   4. safe storage of the drug to prevent accidental overdose.
   A. 1, 2, 3, and 4
   B. 1, 2, and 4
   C. 1, 3, and 4
   D. 2 and 4

9. The nurse is conducting an educational session for the parents of a child diagnosed with varicella. Which one of the following is NOT an appropriate comfort measure to include in this session?
   A. Use Aveeno bath or oatmeal in bath water for added skin comfort.
   B. Use Caladryl lotion on rash to decrease itching.
   C. Use hot bath water to promote skin rash healing.
   D. Keep nails short and smooth to decrease infection from scratching.

10. Which one of the following does the nurse recognize as CONTRAINDICATED in providing comfort measures to children with communicable diseases?
    A. use of acetaminophen for control of elevated temperature in child with varicella
    B. use of imposed bed rest in child with pertussis
    C. use of aspirin to control elevated temperature and/or symptoms in child with varicella
    D. use of lozenges and saline rinses in child 8 years old with sore throat

11. Clinical manifestations differentiate bacterial conjunctivitis from viral conjunctivitis. Which one of the following is present with bacterial conjunctivitis but NOT usually found with viral conjunctivitis?
    A. Child awakens with crusting of eyelids.
    B. Child has increase in watery drainage from eyes.
    C. Child has inflamed conjunctiva.
    D. Child has swollen eyelids.

12. When instructing the parents caring for an infant with conjunctivitis, the nurse will include which one of the following in the plan?
    A. Accumulated secretions are removed by wiping from outer canthus inward.
    B. Hydrogen peroxide placed on cotton swabs is helpful in removing crusts from eyelids.
    C. Compresses of warm tap water are kept in place on the eye to prevent formation of crusting.
    D. Washcloth and towel used by the infant are kept separate and not used by others.

13. Identify the following statements about stomatitis as either TRUE or FALSE.

    _____ Aphthous stomatitis may be associated with mild traumatic injury, allergy, and emotional stress.

    _____ Aphthous stomatitis is painful, small, whitish ulcerations which will heal without complication in 4 to 12 days.

    _____ Herpetic gingivostomatitis is caused by herpes simplex virus, usually type 1.

    _____ Herpetic gingivostomatitis is commonly called "cold sores" or "fever blisters" and may appear in groups or singly.

    _____ Treatment for stomatitis is aimed at relief from complications.

_____ When examining herpetic lesions, the nurse uses his/her uncovered index finger to check for cracks in the skin surface.

14. Anne, an 8-year-old, has been diagnosed with giardiasis. The nurse would expect Anne to have MOST likely presented with which of these signs and symptoms?
    A. diarrhea with blood in the stools
    B. nausea and vomiting with a mild fever
    C. abdominal cramps with intermittent loose stools
    D. weight loss of 5 lb over the last month

15. The nurse is instructing parents on the test tape diagnostic procedure for enterobiasis. Which one of the following is included in the explanation?
    A. Use a flashlight to inspect the anal area while the child sleeps.
    B. Perform the test two days after the child has received the first dose of mebendazole.
    C. Test all members of the family at the same time using frosted tape.
    D. Collect the tape in the morning before the child has a bowel movement or bath.

16. Children with pinworm infections present with the principal symptom of:
    A. perianal itching.
    B. diarrhea with blood.
    C. evidence of small rice-like worms in their stool and urine.
    D. abdominal pain.

17. Reduction of poisonings in children and infants can be accomplished by:
    A. use of child-resistant containers.
    B. educating parents and grandparents to place products out of reach of small children.
    C. educating parents to relocate plants out of reach of infants, toddlers, and small children.
    D. all of the above.

18. The MOST common accidentally ingested medications in children under 6 years of age are:
    A. cold and cough preparations.
    B. analgesics such as acetaminophen and ibuprofen.
    C. hormones such as oral contraception.
    D. antibiotics.

19. The first action parents should be taught to initiate in a poisoning is to:
    A. induce vomiting.
    B. take the child to the family physician's office or emergency center.
    C. call the Poison Control Center.
    D. follow the instructions on the label of the household product.

20. Each toxic ingestion is treated individually. Gastric decontamination is aimed at removing the ingested toxic product by:

    _____

    _____

    _____

    _____

    _____

21. The major principles of emergency treatment for poisoning are _____, _____

_____, _____ _____, _____

_____, and _____ _____ _____.

22. The nurse provides proper administration instructions to parents for ipecac syrup, including which of the following?
    A. Have two doses of emetic in the household for each child.
    B. Administer the emetic within three hours of toxic ingestion.
    C. Never administer out-of-date emetic.
    D. Force fluids and encourage activity after the emetic is administered to facilitate its effectiveness.

23. The nurse does NOT expect to assist in gastric lavage for the treatment of poisoning in which one of the following pediatric patients?
    A. the 8-month-old child admitted to the emergency center who has eaten 8 to 10 holly berries
    B. the 8-year-old child who took three of his mom's birth control pills
    C. the 6-year-old child who has an overdose of a noncorrosive substance and is convulsing
    D. the 13-year-old girl who has an overdose of valium and is comatose

24. Potential causes of heavy metal poisoning in children include _____, _____, and

_____.

25. Identify the following statements as either TRUE or FALSE.

    _____ Asymptomatic young children may have lead levels sufficiently elevated to cause neurologic and intellectual damage.

    _____ The greatest risk of lead poisoning is to poor children under 6 years of age living in urban areas.

    _____ Lead-based paint from old housing remains the most frequent source of lead poisoning in children.

    _____ Lead-containing pottery or leaded dishes do not contribute to lead poisoning because food does not absorb lead.

    _____ Pica is the habitual, purposeful, and compulsive ingestion of nonfood substances.

    _____ The exposure risk is lower for children living in leaded environments whose diet is deficient in iron and calcium and high in fats because the diet slows the absorption of lead.

26. Lead encephalopathy is associated with blood lead concentration of > 100 ug/dl. List four symptoms observed in this condition.

    _____

    _____

    _____

    _____

27. Diagnostic evaluations for lead poisoning include:
    A. blood levels for lead concentration include screening done on finger and heel sticks with blood collected by venipuncture to confirm diagnosis.
    B. recommended universal screening for all children, with children ages 6 to 72 months given priority.
    C. radiographs of the long bones to reveal lead lines caused by deposition of lead.
    D. all of the above.

28. Therapeutic interventions for lead poisoning do NOT include:
    A. removal of the source of lead.
    B. improving nutrition.
    C. using chelation therapy.
    D. administration of dimercaprol intravenously.

29. Match the term with its definition.

    A. child neglect

    B. physical neglect

    C. emotional neglect

    D. emotional abuse

    E. physical abuse

    F. Munchausen syndrome

    _____ deliberate attempt to destroy a child's self-esteem

    _____ failure to meet the child's needs for affection

    _____ deprivation of necessities such as food and clothing

    _____ failure to provide for the child's basic needs and to provide adequate level of care

    _____ deliberate infliction of physical injury on a child

    _____ an illness that one person fabricates or induces in another person

30. Which one of the following parental characteristics does NOT describe abusive parent families?
    A. Teenage mothers are less likely to release frustration by striking out at their children.
    B. Abusive parents have difficulty controlling aggressive impulses.
    C. Free expression of violence is a consistent quality of abusive families.
    D. Abusive families are often more socially isolated and have fewer supportive relationships than nonabusive families.

31. Which one of the following statements is INCORRECT?
    A. The position of the child in the family has little effect on the abusive situation.
    B. One child is usually the victim in an abusive family, and removal of this child often places the other children at risk.
    C. The abusive family environment is one of chronic stress, including problems of divorce, poverty, unemployment, and poor housing.
    D. Child abuse is a problem of all social groups.

32. The nurse is talking with 13-year-old Amy, who has revealed that she is being sexually abused. Which one of the following is a CORRECT guideline for the nurse to utilize?
    A. Promise Amy not to tell what she tells you.
    B. Assure Amy that she will not need to report the abuse.
    C. Avoid using leading statements that can distort Amy's reporting of the problem.
    D. It is okay for the nurse to express anger and shock and to criticize Amy's family.

33. In identification of the abused child, the nurse knows:
    a. incompatibility between the history and the injury is probably the most important criterion on which to base the decision to report suspected abuse.
    B. it is necessary to examine for observable evidence of abuse.
    C. maltreated children rarely betray their parents by admitting to the abuse they received.
    D. all of the above.

❖ *Critical Thinking* ❖
Case Study

Jimmy is a 4-year-old pre-kindergarten student who is brought to the school nurse's office by his teacher. She is concerned because Jimmy has purulent discharge in the corner of both eyes with the conjunctiva appearing inflamed. Jimmy is observed by the school nurse to be wiping his eyes frequently with his hands.

34. Based on the information provided, the nurse suspects the condition that Jimmy has is:
    A. bacterial conjunctivitis.
    B. viral conjunctivitis.
    C. allergic conjunctivitis.
    D. conjunctivitis caused by foreign body.

35. Based on knowledge of communicable disease, the nurse would prioritize which one of the following goals for Jimmy's plan of care?
    A. will not become infected
    B. will not spread disease
    C. will experience minimal discomfort
    D. will maintain skin integrity

36. The school nurse calls Jimmy's parents to request that they come and pick Jimmy up from school. What is the BEST rationale for this action?
    A. Jimmy is tired and needs additional rest because of the infection.
    B. Jimmy is at high risk for spreading the disease because of his age and his inability to wash his hands after touching his eyes.
    C. Jimmy needs immediate medical attention to prevent complications.
    D. The nurse needs to discuss causes of this disease with Jimmy's mother so that its recurrence can be prevented.

37. It is important to include what information in the teaching plan for Jimmy's parents?
    A. Jimmy needs to have his own face cloth and towel.
    B. Eye medication will need to be administered before the eyes are cleaned.
    C. Jimmy cannot return to school until all symptoms have stopped.
    D. Jimmy will need his own eating utensils.

38. The nurse can expect treatment for this disease to include:
    A. use of continuous warm compresses held in place on each infected eye.
    B. application of broad-spectrum topical ophthalmic agents.
    C. oral broad-spectrum antibiotics.
    D. all of the above.

39. The effectiveness of nursing interventions for Jimmy's condition is BEST demonstrated by which one of the following evaluations?
    A. There is no spread of the disease within the school and family.
    B. Parents are able to demonstrate appropriate eye care.
    C. Jimmy reports no eye discomfort.
    D. Jimmy engages in normal activities.

❖ Crossword Puzzle ❖

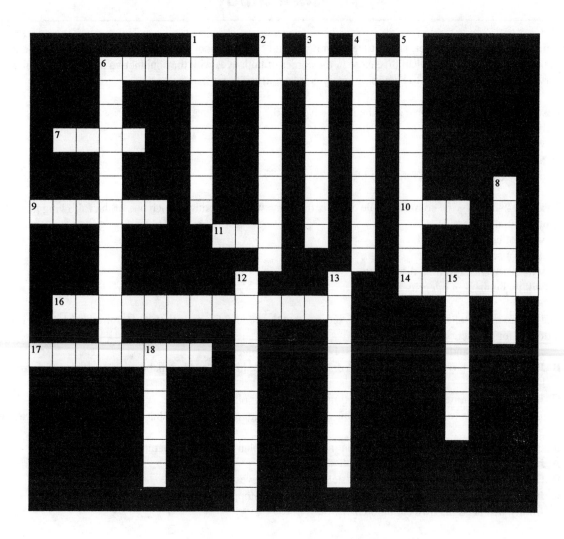

Across

6. Deliberate attempt to destroy or significantly impair a child's physical and/or psychologic development (2 words)
7. Varicella zoster immune globulin
9. Arthropods or other invertebrates that transmit infection
10. British antilewisite
11. Child Protective Services
14. Drug that induces vomiting
16. Older person whose conscious sexual desires or responses are directed toward developmentally immature children or adolescents (2 words)
17. Chronic lead poisoning

Down

1. Dissemination of microbial aerosols
2. Chronic salicylate poisoning
3. Inflamed mucosa with free discharge
4. Restriction of activities of persons who have been exposed to a communicable disease
5. Use of a child for sexual stimulation of an adult or other person (2 words)
6. Indecent exposure
8. Person or animal that harbors an infectious agent without apparent clinical disease
12. Preference of an adult for prepubertal children as a means of achieving sexual excitement
13. Period between early manifestations of disease and overt clinical syndrome
15. Disease occurring regularly within a geographic location
18. Physical sexual activity between family members

❖ CHAPTER 17
Health Promotion of the School-Age Child and Family

1. The middle childhood is also referred to as school-age or the school years. What ages does this period represent?
   A. ages 5 to 13 years
   B. ages 4 to 14 years
   C. ages 6 to 12 years
   D. ages 6 to 16 years

2. Physiologically the middle years begin with _____ and end at

   _____.

3. Which finding should the nurse expect when assessing physical growth in the school-age child?
   A. increase of 2 to 3 kg per year
   B. increase of 3 cm per year
   C. little change in refined coordination
   D. decrease in body fat and muscle tissue

4. Identify the following statements about the school-age child as either TRUE or FALSE.

   _____ In middle childhood there are fewer stomach upsets, better maintenance of blood sugar levels, and an increased stomach capacity.

   _____ Caloric needs are higher in relation to stomach size compared with the needs of preschool years.

   _____ The heart is smaller in relation to the rest of the body during the middle years.

   _____ During the middle years, the immune system develops little immunity to pathogenic microorganisms.

   _____ Back packs are preferred to other book totes during middle years.

   _____ Physical maturity correlates well with emotional and social maturity during the middle years.

5. Early appearance of secondary sex characteristics of girls during preadolescence may be associated with which of the following feelings?
   A. satisfaction with physical appearance and higher self-esteem
   B. increase in self-confidence and a more outgoing personality
   C. dissatisfaction with physical appearance and lower self-esteem
   D. increased substance use and reckless vehicle use

6. Generally, the earliest age at which puberty begins in girls is age _____ and in boys is age

   _____.

7. Middle childhood is the time when children:
   1. learn the value of doing things with others.
   2. learn the benefits derived from division of labor in accomplishing goals.
   3. achieve a sense of industry and accomplishment.
   4. expand interests and engage in tasks that can be carried to completion.
   A. 1, 2, 3, and 4
   B. 1, 3, and 4
   C. 1 and 4
   D. 2 and 3

8. Dillon is a 6-year-old starting in a new neighborhood school. The first day of school he complains of a headache and tearfully tells his mother he does not want to go to school. Dillon's mother takes him to school and the nurse is consulted. The nurse recognizes that Dillon is a slow-to-warm-up child and suggests which one of the following?
   A. Put Dillon in the classroom with the other children and leave him alone.
   B. Insist that Dillon join and lead the class song.
   C. Include Dillon in activities without assigning him tasks until he willingly participates in activities.
   D. Send Dillon home with his mother since he has a headache.

9. During the concrete-operational period of middle childhood, which one of the following is the expected level of cognitive development?
   A. are able to follow directions but unable to verbalize the actions involved in the process
   B. are able to use their thought processes to experience events and actions and make judgments based on what they reason
   C. are able to view from an egocentric outlook that is rigidly developed around the action to be completed
   D. progress from conceptual thinking to perceptual thinking when making judgments

10. Match the term with the accomplishment of cognitive tasks of middle childhood.

    A. conservation   _____ arranging objects according to some ordinal scale

    B. identity   _____ ability to manipulate numbers and to learn the skills of addition, subtraction, multiplication, and division

    C. reversibility
                             _____ ability to group objects according to the attributes they have in
    D. reciprocity   common

    E. classification skills _____ ability to think through an action sequence, anticipate the consequences, and return and rethink the action in a different direction

    F. serialize
                             _____ ability to deal with two dimensions at one time and to comprehend
    G. combinational skills   that a change in one dimension compensates for a change in another

                             _____ able to distinguish a shape change when nothing has been added or subtracted

                             _____ ability to comprehend that physical matter does not appear and disappear by magic

11. A major difference in moral development between young school-age children and older school-age children is BEST described by which one of the following?
    A. Younger children believe that standards of behavior come from within themselves.
    B. Children 6 to 7 years of age know the rules and understand the reasons behind the rules.
    C. Older school-age children are able to judge an act by the intentions that prompted it and not only by the consequences.
    D. all of the above

12. Which one of the following BEST identifies the spiritual development of school-age children?
    A. They have little fear of going to hell for misbehavior.
    B. They begin to learn the difference between the natural and the supernatural.
    C. They petition to God for less tangible rewards.
    D. They view God as a deity with few human traits.

13. Which one of the following would the nurse NOT expect to observe as a characteristic of peer group relationships in 8-year-old Mark?
    A. Mark demonstrates loyalty to the group by adhering to the secret code rules.
    B. Mark demonstrates a greater individual egocentric outlook compared with other peer group members.
    C. Mark is willing to conform to the group's rule of "not talking to girls."
    D. Mark has a best friend within the peer group with whom he shares his secrets.

14. During the school-age years, children learn valuable lessons from age-mates. How is this accomplished?
    A. The child learns to appreciate the varied points of view that are within the peer group.
    B. The child becomes sensitive to the social norms and pressures of the group.
    C. The child's interactions among peers lead to the formation of intimate friendships between same-sex peers.
    D. all of the above

15. With school-age children, the relationship with the family can be observed in which one of the following statements?
    A. Children desire to spend equal time with family and peers.
    B. Children are prepared to reject parental controls.
    C. The group replaces the family as the primary influence in setting standards of behavior and rules.
    D. Children need and want restrictions placed on their behavior by the family.

16. Children's self-concepts are composed of:
    A. their own critical self-assessment.
    B. their interpretations of family members' opinions.
    C. their interpretations of opinions of social contacts outside the family structure.
    D. all of the above.

17. The nurse plans to conduct a sex education class for 10-year-olds. Which information is included in the plan?
    A. Information is presented as a biologic mechanism for the survival of the culture.
    B. Peers supply a large amount of correct sexual information to this age group.
    C. Sexual information supplied by parents usually produces some feelings of guilt and anxiety in children.
    D. Discussions do not include information about both sexes.

18. Team membership characteristics that promote child development during the middle years include which of the following?
    A. Children learn to subordinate personal goals to group goals.
    B. Children learn about division of labor as an effective strategy for the attainment of a goal.
    C. Team play helps children to learn about the nature of competition and the importance of winning.
    D. all of the above

19. The factor that MOST influences the amount and manner of discipline and limit-setting imposed on school-age children is:
    A. the age of the parent.
    B. the education of the parent.
    C. response of the child to rewards and punishments.
    D. the ability of the parent to communicate with the school system.

20. To assist school-age children in coping with stress in their lives, the nurse should:
    1. be able to recognize signs that indicate the child is undergoing stress.
    2. teach the child how to recognize signs of stress in herself/himself.
    3. help the child plan a means for dealing with any stress through problem solving.
    4. reassure the child that the stress is only temporary.
    A. 1, 2, 3, and 4
    B. 1, 2, and 3
    C. 1, 2, and 4
    D. 1 and 3

21. Which one of the following statements, describing fears in the school-age child, is TRUE?
    A. School-age children are increasingly fearful for body safety.
    B. Most of the new fears that trouble school-age children are related to school and family.
    C. School-age children should be encouraged to hide their fears to prevent ridicule by their peers.
    D. School-age children with numerous fears need continuous protective behavior by parents to eliminate these fears.

22. By the end of middle childhood, children should be able to assume personal responsibility for self-care in the areas of

    _____, _____, _____, _____,

    _____, and _____.

23. Sleep problems in the school-age child are often demonstrated by:
    A. delaying tactics because they do not wish to go to bed.
    B. the occurrence of night terrors that awaken the child during the night.
    C. the development of somatic illness that awakens the child during the night.
    D. the increasing need for larger amounts of sleep time compared with preschool and adolescence.

24. The nurse is planning to advise a school-age child's parents about appropriate physical activity for their child. Which fact does the nurse include?
    A. School-age children have the same stamina and control as 15-year-old teens.
    B. School-age children are prepared for participation in strenuous competitive athletics.
    C. Activities that promote coordination in the school-age child include running and skipping rope.
    D. Most children need continued encouragement to engage in physical activity.

25. List four components included in the content of school health services.

    _____

    _____

    _____

    _____

26. The nurse is planning an educational session for a group of 9-year-olds and their parents which is aimed at decreasing injuries and accidents among this group. The nurse would BEST accomplish this goal by including what topics in the educational session?
    A. safety rules when dealing with fire to prevent burns
    B. safety rules when dealing with toxic substances to prevent poisonings
    C. pedestrian safety rules and skills training programs to prevent motor vehicle accidents
    D. reviewing the rules for the use of all-terrain vehicles and encouraging their use only with supervision

❖ *Critical Thinking* ❖
Case Study

Allen Thomas, age 9, is taken to the clinic by his mother for a school physical examination. Allen's mother is concerned because Allen wants to join the school soccer team this year. On physical examination, the nurse discovers that since last year Allen has had an increase of 2 inches in height and has gained 10 pounds. Health history is unchanged from the previous year. Allen tells the nurse that he rides his bike more now than last year because he has a new "best friend" to go riding with.

27. Based on the above information, the nurse should expand assessment with Allen in which of the following areas at this visit?
    1. his diet
    2. his knowledge and use of safety precautions when riding his bike
    3. his hygiene habits
    4. his reasons for wanting to play soccer
    A. 1, 2, and 3
    B. 2 and 4
    C. 1 and 2
    D. 1 and 4

28. Which of the following would be the nurse's BEST response to the mother's concern about Allen playing soccer?
    A. "Allen is healthy, and playing soccer will allow him to increase strength and develop motor skill performance."
    B. "Allen is overweight for his age and should be encouraged to ride his bike less. Soccer is a better activity for him since it will help decrease his weight."
    C. "Allen is still too young to participate in strenuous sports like soccer. He should be able to participate in another year."
    D. "Let Allen play what he wants to. You worry too much about his activities."

29. Based on the above information, the nurse plans an educational session for Allen and his mother. The knowledge deficit that the nurse is MOST likely to have identified with this family is:
    A. altered nutrition related to improper dietary habits.
    B. altered nutrition: less than body requirements.
    C. lack of proper physical activity related to bike riding.
    D. improper parenting skills related to overprotective mother.

30. Mrs. Thomas asks the nurse how she can foster Allen's development. What should be the response by the nurse?
    A. "Don't interfere with Allen as long as he is doing well in school."
    B. "Give Allen recognition and positive feedback for his accomplishments."
    C. "Always point out to Allen how he incorrectly performs tasks so that he can improve his accomplishments."
    D. "Try not to set rules for Allen. He needs to set his own limits during this period of development."

❖ Crossword Puzzle ❖

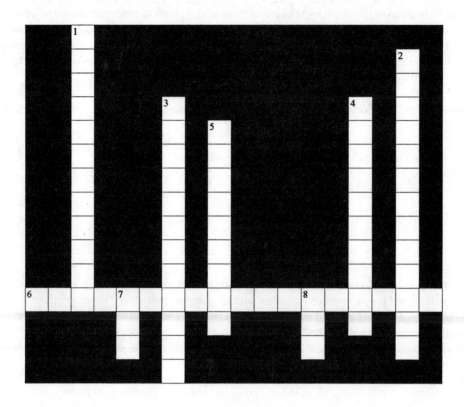

Across

6. More logical thought about real objects and experiences (2 words)

Down

1. Thinking on a symbolic level; unable to use cognitive operations
2. Approximately two years during which preliminary physical changes leading to sexual maturity take place
3. Recognition that properties of an object or substance do not change when its appearance is superficially altered
4. The tendency to view the world from one's own perspective
5. An action performed on an object or set of objects
7. Rapid eye movement
8. All-terrain vehicle

❖ CHAPTER 18
Health Problems of Middle Childhood

1. Functions performed by the skin do NOT include:
   A. protection.
   B. heat regulation.
   C. sensation.
   D. nutrition.

2. The three layers of the skin are the _____, _____, and _____ tissue.

3. Match the term related to assessment of the skin with its definition.

   A. pruritus   _____ reddened area caused by increased amounts of blood

   B. anesthesia   _____ localized purple discolorations

   C. hyperesthesia   _____ pinpoint, tiny, circumscribed hemorrhagic spots

   D. paresthesia   _____ skin changes caused by some causative factor to produce macules, papules, or vesicles

   E. erythema

   F. ecchymoses   _____ changes related to rubbing, scratching, or medication

                            _____ whether the pattern is localized or generalized

   G. petechiae   _____ the size and shape of the lesions or the group of lesions

   H. primary lesions

                            _____ itching

   I. secondary lesions

                            _____ excessive sensitiveness

   J. distribution   _____ absence of sensation

   K. configuration   _____ abnormal sensation

4. Match the term related to wounds with its definition.

A. acute   _____ accidental cut, either torn or jagged edges

B. chronic   _____ disruption of the skin that extends into the underlying tissue or into a body cavity

C. pressure ulcer

      _____ heals uneventfully within the usual time frame

D. abrasion

      _____ does not heal in the expected time frame and can be associated with complications

E. evulsion

F. laceration   _____ removal of the superficial layers of skin by scraping

G. incision   _____ often becomes chronic skin injury and is a localized area of cellular necrosis

H. penetrating   _____ forcible pulling out or extraction of tissue

I. puncture   _____ wound with opening that is small compared with depth

      _____ division of the skin made with a sharp object

5. During wound healing, immature connective tissue cells migrate to the healing site and begin to secrete collagen into the meshwork spaces. What is this phase called?
   A. scar contracture
   B. inflammation
   C. fibroplasia
   D. scar maturation

6. Mary, age 7, fell and sustained a deep laceration to her chin. She was taken to the emergency center where the laceration was sutured with the edges well approximated. The nurse expects the repair healing to take place by:
   A. primary intention.
   B. secondary intention.
   C. tertiary intention.
   D. all of the above.

7. The nurse recognizes that a factor that is NOT indicated for use in promoting wound healing is:
   A. nutrition with sufficient protein, calories, vitamin C, and zinc.
   B. irrigation of wounds with normal saline.
   C. application of povidone-iodine daily.
   D. application of an occlusive dressing.

8. Skin disorder assessment includes the objective data collected by inspection and palpation. Which one of the following is NOT objective data?
   A. The lesion has an increased erythema margin edge.
   B. The rash appears as macules and papules.
   C. The lesion is painful and itches.
   D. The lesion is moist.

9. Care of bacterial skin infections in children may include all of the following EXCEPT:
   A. good handwashing.
   B. keeping the fingernails short.
   C. puncturing the surface of the pustule.
   D. application of topical antibiotics.

10. Which one of the following is a fungal infection that lives on the skin?
    A. tinea corporis
    B. herpes simplex type 1
    C. scabies
    D. warts

11. Which one of the following statements about scabies is INCORRECT?
    A. Clinical manifestations include intense pruritus, especially at night, and papules, burrows, or vesicles on inter-digital surfaces.
    B. Treatment is the application of 1% Kwell or 5% Elimite for all family members.
    C. After treatment, all previously worn clothing is washed in very hot water and ironed.
    D. The rash and itching will be eliminated immediately after treatment.

12. The nurse is instructing Angie's parents about using the prescribed Kwell shampoo for pediculosis. Which one of the following is included in these instructions?
    A. The shampoo will be used only once and left on for only 4 hours.
    B. The shampoo is toxic when used on children under 2 years of age.
    C. The shampoo kills the lice and nits on contact.
    D. The lice jump and fly from one person to another.

13. Children with lyme disease do NOT present with which of the following signs and symptoms?
    A. small erythematous papule that has a circumferential ring with a raised, edematous doughnut-like border
    B. multiple, small secondary annular lesions with indurated centers on the palms and soles
    C. flu-like symptoms of headache, malaise, lymphadenopathy
    D. abdominal pain, splenomegaly, fatigue, anorexia

14. Billy has come in contact with poison ivy on a school picnic. The BEST intervention for the nurse to implement at this time is:
    A. washing the area with a strong soap and water solution.
    B. applying Calamine lotion to the area.
    C. preventing spread by instructing Billy not to scratch the lesions.
    D. washing the area with alcohol.

15. When advising parents about the use of sunscreen for their children, the nurse should tell them that:
    A. a waterproof sunscreen with a minimum 15 SPF is recommended for children.
    B. the lower the number of SPF, the higher the protection.
    C. sunscreens are not as effective as sun blockers.
    D. the sunscreen should be applied one hour before the child is allowed in the sun.

16. In caring for the child with frostbite, the nurse remembers that:
    A. slow thawing is associated with less tissue necrosis.
    B. the frostbitten part appears white or blanched, feels solid, and is without sensation.
    C. rewarming produces a small return of sensation with a small amount of pain.
    D. rewarming is accomplished by rubbing the injured tissue.

17. Skin disorders related to drug sensitivity include:
    A. erythema multiform.
    B. Stevens-Johnson syndrome.
    C. toxic epidermal necrolysis.
    D. all of the above.

18. Neurofibromatosis is:
    A. an autosomal dominant genetic disorder.
    B. suspected when the 5-year-old child presents with six or more cafe-au-lait spots larger than 5 mm in diameter.
    C. suspected when the infant develops axillary or inguinal freckling.
    D. all of the above.

19. The MOST effective method for tick removal in a child is to:
    A. use curved forceps and pull straight up with a steady, even pressure.
    B. apply mineral oil to the back of the tick and wait for it to back out.
    C. use the fingers to pull the tick out with a straight, steady, even pressure.
    D. place a hot match on the back of the tick and pick it up with gloved hands when the tick falls off.

20. Dog bites in children:
    A. occur most often in girls over 4 years of age.
    B. occur most often in children less than 4 years of age.
    C. occur most often from stray dogs.
    D. occur most often in school yards and neighborhood parks.

21. The MOST common cause of malocclusion is:
    A. thumb-sucking.
    B. tongue thrusting.
    C. heredity.
    D. abnormal growth patterns.

22. Emergency care for tooth evulsion includes:
    A. replanting the tooth after bleeding has stopped.
    B. storing the tooth in tap water until it and the child can be transported to the dentist.
    C. holding the tooth by the root.
    D. rinsing the dirty tooth with milk before replanting.

23. The major nursing consideration in assisting the family of a child with nocturnal enuresis is to prevent the child from developing alterations in:
    A. body image.
    B. self-esteem.
    C. autonomy.
    D. peer acceptance.

24. The nurse is assisting the family of a child with a history of encopresis. Which one of the following should be included in the nurse's discussion with this family?
    A. Instruct the parents to sit the child on the toilet at twice-daily routine intervals.
    B. Instruct the parents that the child will probably need to have daily enemas for the next year.
    C. Suggest the use of stimulant cathartics weekly.
    D. Reassure the family that most problems resolve successfully, with some relapses during periods of stress

25. Barbara has been diagnosed with attention-deficit hyperactivity disorder and placed on methylphenidate (Ritalin) by her physician. Which one of the following statements, if made by the nurse to Barbara's parents, is CORRECT?
    A. "Methylphenidate is preferred because of its less marked effect on growth hormones."
    B. "Dosage is usually unchanged until adolescence."
    C. "This medication takes two to three weeks to achieve an effect."
    D. "Barbara's appetite will be increased with this drug."

26. Therapeutic management for tics in children primarily consists of:
    A. behavioral modification to teach the child to suppress the tic disorder.
    B. administration of haloperidol to suppress the tic disorder.
    C. support for the child and family with reassurance about the prognosis.
    D. genetic counseling for the parents.

27. Identify the following statements as either TRUE or FALSE.

    _____ School phobia is more common in boys than in girls.

    _____ School-phobia children are correctly viewed as delinquent children.

_____ A frequent source of fear in school phobia is separation anxiety based on a strong dependent relationship between the mother and the child.

_____ The primary goal for the child with school phobia is to return the child to school.

_____ Prevention of dependency problems in childhood is based on encouraging independence at appropriate times during infancy and early childhood.

_____ Recurrent abdominal pain of childhood is defined as three or more separate episodes of abdominal pain during a three-month period.

_____ Children at risk for recurrent abdominal pain tend to be high achievers with great personal goals or children whose parents have unusually high expectations.

_____ Depressed children usually exhibit low-esteem, think of themselves as hopeless, and explain negative events in terms of their personal shortcomings.

_____ Three risk factors identified for childhood schizophrenia are genetic characteristics, gestational and birth complications, and winter birth.

❖ Critical Thinking ❖
Case Study

Carol, age 9, went on a picnic yesterday with her family. Today she returns to school and is showing her classmates several leaves that she collected yesterday on her picnic. The teacher notes that three of the leaves are poison ivy. The teacher takes Carol to the school nurse because of a rash that has developed on Carol's arms and legs. Carol tells the nurse that the rash is "very itchy."

28. The nurse completes a diagnostic assessment of the skin rash to include a complete history and physical examination. The nurse knows that this history should include:
    A. inspection of the rash including size and shape of lesions.
    B. symptoms, past and recent exposure to causative agents, medications taken, and history of previous similar rashes.
    C. palpation of the rash for increased heat, edema, and tenderness.
    D. skin scrapings from the site for microscopic examination.

29. The primary action the school nurse should take at this time is:
    A. call Carol's parents to pick her up at school. Isolate Carol from other classmates until her parents arrive.
    B. give the poison ivy leaves to the school janitor so that they can be destroyed in the school incinerator.
    C. instruct the teacher to make sure all classmates who had contact with the poison ivy plant wash these areas with mild soap and water or alcohol.
    D. reassure Carol that everything is going to be fine, apply Calamine lotion to Carol's rash, and instruct Carol not to scratch the rash.

30. The BEST nursing diagnosis for Carol at this time would be:
    A. impaired skin integrity related to environmental factors.
    B. high risk for infection related to presence of infectious organisms.
    C. pain related to skin lesions.
    D. body image disturbance related to presence of rash.

31. Goals for Carol will include which of the following?
    A. Carol will not experience secondary damage, such as infection, from scratching.
    B. Carol will demonstrate acceptable levels of comfort from itching.
    C. Carol will be able to recognize and avoid precipitating agent in the future.
    D. all of the above

❖ Crossword Puzzle ❖

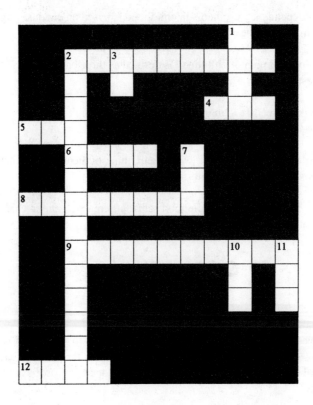

Across

2. Pinpoint spots in the superficial layers of the epidermis
4. Recurrent abdominal pain
5. Erythema chronicum migrans
6. Attention-deficit hyperactivity disorder
8. A reddened area caused by increased amounts of oxygenated blood in the dermal vasculature
9. Bruises
12. Post-traumatic stress disorder

Down

1. p-aminobenzoic acid
2. Skin changes produced by some causative factor (2 words)
3. Tourette syndrome
7. Ultraviolet A
10. Stevens-Johnson syndrome
11. Sun protection factor

❖ CHAPTER 19
Health Promotion of the Adolescent and Family

1. In the female adolescent who has reached puberty, the luteinizing hormone (LH) initiates which of the following actions?
   A. ovulation
   B. formation of the corpus luteum
   C. progesterone production
   D. all of the above

2. The hormone in the female that causes growth and development of the vagina, uterus, and fallopian tubes as well as breast enlargement is:
   A. estrogen.
   B. progesterone.
   C. follicle-stimulating hormone.
   D. luteinizing hormone.

3. Identify the following statements regarding adolescence as either TRUE or FALSE.

   _____ The adolescent is considered potentially fertile from the first menstrual period or first ejaculation.

   _____ Development of secondary sexual characteristics occurs in a predictable sequence.

   _____ The Tanner developmental stages is a classification system based on maturity of secondary sex characteristics that can be utilized when assessing adolescent growth.

   _____ Hypothalamic-pituitary-gonadal system is maintained in an active state throughout childhood because of the low secretion of gonadotropin-releasing hormone.

   _____ The development of small bud of breast tissue is the earliest, most easily visible change of puberty.

   _____ The average age for beginning menstruation is 13.

4. Julie, 12 years old, is brought to the nurse practitioner's office by her mother. Julie has started to develop breast tissue and some pubic hair. Both the mother and Julie are concerned because Julie has been having increased vaginal discharge. Julie tells the nurse, "I wash my private area every day, but I still have fluid that comes out." What is the nurse's BEST response?
   A. "It sounds as if you have an infection. We'll have the nurse practitioner check you to see what is causing this discharge."
   B. "Have you been using soap when you wash?"
   C. "This sounds like a normal discharge that happens to all girls as they start to mature. It is a sign your body is preparing for your periods to begin."
   D. "This is probably not related to hygiene. Are you concerned that this discharge might be causing an odor?"

5. Girls may be considered to have _____ _____ if breast development has not occurred by age 13 or if menarche has not occurred by age 13.

6. The first pubescent change in boys is:
   A. appearance of pubic hair.
   B. testicular enlargement with thinning, reddening, and increased looseness of the scrotum.
   C. penile enlargement.
   D. temporary breast enlargement and tenderness.

7. Tommy is brought in by his father for his yearly physical. On examination, the nurse notes that since last year Tommy has developed pubic hair, testicular enlargement, and related scrotal changes. In planning anticipatory guidance, the nurse recognizes that which one of the following subjects would BEST be discussed with Tommy as soon as possible?
   A. nocturnal emission
   B. sexually transmitted disease prevention
   C. pregnancy prevention
   D. hygiene needs

8. The _____ _____ refers to the increased growth of muscles, skeleton, and internal organs that peaks during puberty.

9. Which one of the following statements about pattern of growth during adolescence is TRUE?
   A. Knowing the correct sequence of the growth pattern is useful only when assessing abnormal growth patterns versus normal growth patterns.
   B. Girls usually begin puberty and reach maturity about two years earlier than boys.
   C. Girls and boys start an increase of muscle mass during early puberty that lasts throughout adolescence.
   D. Girls and boys have an increase in linear growth that begins for both during midpuberty.

10. On the average, girls gain _____ to _____ inches in height and _____ to _____ pounds during adolescence, while

    boys gain _____ to _____ inches and _____ to _____ pounds.

11. Which one of the following BEST describes the formal operational thinking that occurs between the ages of 11 and 14 years?
    A. Thought process includes thinking in concrete terms.
    B. Thought process includes information obtained from the environment and peers.
    C. Thought process includes thinking in abstract terms, possibilities, and hypotheses.
    D. all of the above

12. Jimmy, a 13-year-old, is sent to the school nurse because he and some of his peers were caught chewing tobacco while playing baseball. The nurse knows that the BEST way to influence Jimmy's behavior for health promotion would be which of the following?
    A. Tell Jimmy that he will be suspended from school if he continues to chew the tobacco.
    B. Show Jimmy pictures of oral cancers caused by chewing tobacco.
    C. Tell Jimmy about the dangers of chewing tobacco and stress the fact that girls do not like boys who chew tobacco.
    D. Arrange for a local baseball hero to talk with Jimmy and his friends to stress that he does not use chewing tobacco, his friends do not chew tobacco, and chewing tobacco causes ugly teeth.

13. Adolescent egocentrism may lead to a pattern of personal fable. An example of a personal fable is:
    A. "Everyone is coming to the play just to see me."
    B. "Mary Sue got pregnant, but it won't happen to me."
    C. "I hate taking my clothes off for gym class because everyone stares at me."
    D. "Mary is very envious of how I dress."

14. According to Erikson, a key to identity achievement in adolescence is BEST described as:
    A. related to the adolescent's interactions with others that serves as a mirror reflecting information back to the adolescent.
    B. linked to the role he/she plays within the family.
    C. related to the adolescent's acceptance of parental guidelines.
    D. related to the adolescent's ability to complete his/her plans for future accomplishments.

15. The formation of sexual identity development during adolescence usually involves which of the following?
    A. forming close friendships with same-sex peers during early adolescence
    B. developing intimate relationships with members of the opposite sex during the later part of adolescence
    C. developing emotional and social identities separate from those of families
    D. all of the above

16. Nationally, what percentage of boys and girls have had sexual intercourse by the age of 18?
    A. 45% of boys and 65% of girls
    B. 80% of boys and 20% of girls
    C. 45% of girls and 65% of boys
    D. 80% of girls and 20% of boys

17. Intimate relationships are NOT characterized by which one of the following?
    A. concern for each other's well-being
    B. sharing of sexual intimacy
    C. a willingness to disclose private, sensitive topics
    D. sharing of common interests and activities

18. Changes in family structure and parent employment have resulted in certain changes for adolescents, including:
    A. adolescents having more time unsupervised by adults.
    B. adolescents having more time for communication and intimacy with parents.
    C. adolescents having less time to spend with peers.
    D. adolescents requiring more supervision by outside family members.

19. Adolescents who feel close to their parents show:
    1. more positive psychosocial development.
    2. greater behavioral competence.
    3. less susceptibility to negative peer pressure.
    4. lower tendencies to be involved in risk-taking behaviors.
    A. 1, 3, and 4
    B. 1 and 2
    C. 3 and 4
    D. 1, 2, 3, and 4

20. During adolescence, advances in cognitive development bring which one of the following changes?
    A. Their beliefs become more concrete and less rooted in general ideologic principles.
    B. They show an increasing emotional understanding and acceptance of parents' beliefs as their own.
    C. They encounter few new situations or opportunities for decisions because of their past experiences.
    D. They develop a personal value system distinct from that of significant adults in their lives.

21. Compared with children, adolescent peer groups are:
    A. more likely in girls.
    B. less autonomous.
    C. less likely to influence members' socialization roles.
    D. more likely to require parental supervision.

22. The timing of transition from elementary school to junior high has proven to be of significance for the adolescent. Students age 12 or 13 who are transferred to junior high for 7th grade are BEST described by which one of the following?
    A. more positive self-esteem and leadership, especially among girls
    B. less positive self-esteem and leadership, especially among girls
    C. higher grade point averages
    D. less likely to be victims of robbery, beatings, or threats

23. The primary cause of mortality during adolescence is:
    A. drownings.
    B. homicides.
    C. suicides.
    D. motor vehicle crashes.

24. Major causes of morbidity during adolescence include:
    A. motor vehicle injuries.
    B. sexually transmitted diseases.
    C. substance abuse.
    D. all of the above.

25. To BEST effect adolescent health promotion activity, the nurse should incorporate which one of the following in the plan?
    A. the adolescent's definition of health
    B. the adolescent's past health promotion activities
    C. a complete assessment of the adolescent's past medical treatment
    D. a complete physical examination

26. Health concerns consistent with middle adolescents include:
    A. school performance.
    B. emotional health issues.
    C. physical appearance.
    D. future career or employment.

27. Adolescents are more likely to participate in health care services when:
    A. they feel confidentiality about sexual activity and substance abuse will be maintained.
    B. they see the health care provider as caring and respectful.
    C. the family has adequate financial resources, including health insurance.
    D. all of the above

28. Identify the following statements as either TRUE or FALSE.

    _____ Protective factors that characterize adolescents who cope successfully with adverse life situations include the ability to adapt to new persons and situations.

    _____ The nurse involved with adolescent health promotion should plan interventions that decrease exposures to stressful life events and increase sources of emotional support.

    _____ The most successful adolescent health promotion programs are aimed at single issues presented with a focused educational approach.

    _____ When interviewing adolescents, the nurse begins with questions of a less sensitive nature and ends with those of a more sensitive nature.

    _____ For black teens the most likely cause of death is homicide.

29. Adolescent girls of low socioeconomic status are particularly at risk for dietary deficiencies of:
    1. calories.
    2. sodium.
    3. calcium.
    4. folic acid.
    5. iron.
    A. 1, 2, and 3
    B. 2, 3, 4, and 5
    C. 3, 4, and 5
    D. 1, 3, and 5

❖ Critical Thinking ❖
Case Study

Carol, a 16-year-old, visits the nurse practitioner for a routine checkup. She is an A and B student in school and a member of the girls' drill team. Carol matured early and started to menstruate at the age of 10. Her menses are now regular. Carol has a boyfriend and has been dating since the age of 13. She tells the nurse she has no specific concerns.

30. Based on risk factors associated with teens Carol's age, the nurse recognizes which one of the following as the MOST important to discuss with Carol at this visit?
    A. Carol's perception and concerns about health
    B. Carol's nutritional habits
    C. Carol's sexual activity
    D. Carol's relationship with her family

31. The nurse establishes a trusting relationship with Carol, and Carol admits to having been sexually active with five boys since she started dating. Besides educating Carol on the risks of sexually transmitted diseases and pregnancy, which one of the following is MOST important for the nurse to include in the plan of care for Carol at this time?
    A. Discuss with Carol how she can tell her parents about her sexual activity.
    B. Explore possible reasons for Carol's behavior with her.
    C. Assess Carol's immunization status for hepatitis B.
    D. Assess how Carol feels about the possibility of getting pregnant.

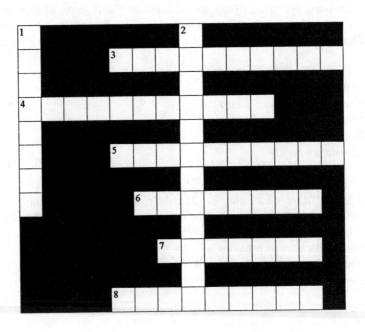

Across

3. Pubertal changes caused by increased secretion of androgenic hormones or their precursors
4. Maturational process initiated by pubertal changes
5. Sexual attraction to persons of the same sex
6. The condition of being a specific person
7. Achievement of sexual maturity
8. Beginning of breast development in the female

Down

1. Establishment of menstrual function
2. Sexual attraction to persons of the opposite sex

❖ CHAPTER 20
Physical Health Problems of Adolescence

1. The type of lesions seen in acne that are more prone to cause scarring are:
   A. non-inflamed lesions.
   B. closed comedones.
   C. inflamed lesions.
   D. blackheads.

2. Nancy, age 16 years, presents to the nurse because of acne on her face, shoulders, and neck areas. After talking with Nancy, the nurse makes a nursing diagnosis of knowledge deficit related to proper skin care. Which one of the following would the nurse include in the instruction plan for Nancy?
   A. Wash the areas vigorously with antibacterial soap.
   B. Brush the hair down on the forehead to conceal the acne areas.
   C. Avoid the use of all cosmetics.
   D. Gently wash the areas with a mild soap once or twice daily.

3. The practitioner has prescribed Retin-A for Nancy's acne, and Nancy returns for a follow-up visit after one month of treatment. During the nursing assessment, Nancy tells the nurse that she has "done everything" she was told to do and asks, "Why is my acne no better?" The nurse's BEST reply is:
   A. "Since the medication prevents the formation of new comedones, it will take two to three months for improvement to be obvious."
   B. "You must not be using the medication right. Show me how you apply it to your face."
   C. "Acne is caused by dirt or oil on the surface of the skin. You will need to increase the number of times you wash these areas each day."
   D. "You will probably need to ask the practitioner about changing your medicine as soon as possible."

4. The MOST common solid tumor in males 15 to 34 years of age is:
   A. varicocele.
   B. testicular torsion.
   C. priapism.
   D. testicular cancer.

5. The adolescent with testicular cancer is MOST likely to present with which one of the following signs and symptoms?
   A. tender, painful swelling of the testes
   B. a mass in the posterior aspect of the scrotum that transilluminates
   C. a heavy, hard, painless mass palpable on the anterior or lateral surface of the testicle
   D. asymptomatic scrotal mass that aches, especially after exercise or penile erection

6. In teaching the adolescent male how to perform testicular self-examination, the nurse includes which of the following instructions?
   A. Perform the procedure once a month after a warm shower.
   B. A raised swelling palpated on the superior aspect of the testicle indicates an abnormality.
   C. Use the second and third fingers on each hand, holding each testicle between the fingers while it is palpated with the other fingers.
   D. all of the above

7. The nurse knows that which of the following adolescent females should be scheduled for her first pelvic examination?
   A. the 18-year-old who has not become sexually active
   B. the adolescent who has been menstruating for two years and has severe dysmenorrhea that is unrelieved by medication
   C. the adolescent who wants to start birth control pills
   D. all of the above

8. Match the term with its definition. (Terms may be used more than once.)

   A. varicocele   _____ breast enlargement that occurs during puberty

   B. epididymitis   _____ is palpated as a wormlike mass above the testicle that becomes smaller in
                                     size when the adolescent lies down

   C. testicular torsion
                            _____ treatment includes assurance to the adolescent that the disease is benign and
   D. gynecomastia   temporary and occurs in about 50% of his peers

                            _____ inflammation that is a result of either infection or local trauma

                            _____ the testis hangs free from its vascular structure; results in partial or complete
                                     venous occlusion

                            _____ presents with unilateral scrotal pain, redness, and swelling; may have urethral
                                     discharge, dysuria, fever, and pyuria; treatment is with antibiotics

                            _____ presents with scrotum that is swollen, painful, red, and warm; adolescent
                                     will have pain radiating to groin, with nausea, vomiting, and abdominal
                                     pain; fever and urinary symptoms are usually not present; treatment is im-
                                     mediate surgery

9. _____ _____ is defined as an absence of menses by age 16 when there are nor-

   mal secondary sexual characteristics. _____ _____ is defined as an absence of
   menses for three to six months in a previously menstruating female when pregnancy has been excluded.

10. The treatment of choice for an adolescent with dysmenorrhea is:
    A. acetaminophen.
    B. oral contraceptives.
    C. nonsteroidal antiinflammatory drugs.
    D. estrogen suppression drugs.

11. Adverse effects of exercise on an adolescent's reproductive cycle may include:
    A. delayed menarche.
    B. anovulation associated with dysfunctional uterine bleeding.
    C. amenorrhea.
    D. all of the above.

12. Match the term with its description.

A. dysmenorrhea

B. premenstrual syndrome

C. endometriosis

D. dysfunctional uterine bleeding

E. vaginitis candidiasis

F. pelvic inflammatory disease

G. trichomonas vaginalis

_____ It has more than 100 associated physical, psychologic, and behavioral symptoms.

_____ It may be caused by the presence of endometrial tissue outside the uterine cavity.

_____ abnormal vaginal bleeding usually associated with anovulation

_____ painful menses

_____ infection of the upper genital tract commonly caused by gonorrhea or chlamydia

_____ It may present with vaginal pruritus and dysuria and is not an STD.

_____ anaerobic parasitic protozoan; is an STD

13. Shirley, age 17, has been diagnosed with pelvic inflammatory disease caused by gonorrhea. The nurse can expect treatment to include which one of the following?
    A. Shirley will be hospitalized to ensure compliance with treatment.
    B. Shirley will be given rocephin intramuscularly and additional oral antibiotics as outpatient treatment.
    C. No treatment of Shirley's partner will be necessary.
    D. Shirley will be placed on oral contraceptives.

14. Adolescent girls have a higher rate of preterm labor than women of other age groups. A possible reason for this is:
    A. the incomplete growth and physiologic immaturity of the adolescent.
    B. the lack of educational resources available to the adolescent.
    C. the irregularity of the menstrual cycle.
    D. the high incidence of pelvic inflammatory disease among this group.

15. The nurse knows that which of the following adolescents would be at high risk for premarital pregnancy?
    A. those who have early initiation of sexual activity
    B. the adolescent who does not use a reliable method of contraception regularly
    C. the adolescent of African-American or Hispanic culture
    D. all of the above

16. Infants of adolescents are at risk because:
    A. teenage mothers often neglect their infants, leaving them for long periods with grandparents.
    B. teenage mothers supply excessive amounts of cognitive stimulation to their infants.
    C. adolescents are less sensitive to their infant's cues.
    D. adolescents are less likely to treat their infants as love objects or playthings.

17. The first goal in the nursing care of the pregnant teenager is:
    A. to arrange for the pregnant teen to register for food supplement programs to ensure proper nutrition.
    B. to assist the pregnant teen in obtaining prenatal care.
    C. to involve the boyfriend and parents in the pregnancy so that the pregnant teen will have support during her pregnancy.
    D. to educate the pregnant teen regarding child care.

18. Children of teenage mothers experience:
    A. more academic difficulties.
    B. more problems with self-esteem.
    C. less emotional misbehavior.
    D. greater physical disability during childhood.

19. Emily is an unmarried 17-year-old who is six weeks pregnant and who has decided to have an abortion. One nursing action used to assist Emily would be:
    A. explaining to Emily that it is wrong for her to have an abortion and arranging for Emily to visit an adoption center.
    B. referral of Emily to an appropriate abortion agency when Emily is four months pregnant.
    C. providing Emily with relaxation strategies to be used during the procedure.
    D. calling Emily's parents so that they can be present for the abortion.

20. In discussing prevention of sexually transmitted diseases, the nurse tells the adolescent that which one of the following is MOST effective?
    A. birth control pills
    B. Norplant
    C. spermicides
    D. condoms

21. Nancy, age 17, is brought to the family planning clinic by her mother for birth control. Which one of the following does the nurse recognize as being MOST important to include in the plan with Nancy at this time?
    A. discussion of the effectiveness rates for various methods and importance of compliance
    B. including Nancy's partner in the discussions
    C. discussion of Nancy's perception of likelihood of getting pregnant and her desire to prevent pregnancy versus her desire for pregnancy
    D. cost of the various methods of contraception

22. Which of the following is CONTRAINDICATED as a method of birth control in Nancy?
    A. intrauterine device
    B. sponge
    C. Depo-Provera
    D. diaphragm

23. Rape victims display a variety of manifestations. Which of the following might the nurse see in 16-year-old Sally as she arrives at the emergency center for treatment?
    A. hysterical crying or giggling
    B. calm and controlled behavior
    C. anger and rage alternating with helplessness and agitation
    D. all of the above

24. The primary goal of nursing care for the adolescent rape victim is:
    A. not to inflict further stress on the victim.
    B. obtaining a complete history of the incident.
    C. assisting in the physical examination.
    D. notifying the police and the parents of the victim before proceeding with assessment.

25. Identify the following statements about sexually transmitted diseases in adolescence as either TRUE or FALSE.

    _____ Adolescent females are at a lower risk for chlamydia and human papillomavirus because of the immature adolescent endocervix.

    _____ In the adolescent, the immune system provides excellent localized antibody response to infectious agents at the cervical level.

    _____ Research has demonstrated that as the use of hormonal contraception increases, the use of condoms declines among adolescents.

    _____ Adolescents ages 15 to 19 have the highest overall incidence of gonococcal infection compared with other age groups.

_____ Symptoms of gonorrhea can occur 1 day to 16 days after sexual contact, or there may be an absence of all symptoms.

_____ Gonorrhea is seen in the prepubescent adolescent as vulvovaginitis and in the postpubescent female as a urogenital infection involving the cervix.

_____ Collection of a specimen from the cervix for gonorrhea must be delayed until the adolescent is not on her menses.

_____ Treatment for gonorrhea includes both the partner and the client and provides lifelong immunity.

26. Therapeutic management for chlamydia includes:
    A. doxycycline, 100 mg bid for seven days in the pregnant adolescent and her partner.
    B. intramuscular injection of rocephin 125 mg for the client and partner.
    C. intramuscular injection of penicillin 2.4 million units for the client and partner.
    D. azithromycin 1 gram po in a single dose for the client and her partner.

27. The MOST common STD in the United States is _____. These individu-

    als are at risk for development of _____ _____ and _____.

28. One STD for which there is now immunization recommended for all adolescents is:
    A. human immunodeficiency virus.
    B. hepatitis B virus.
    C. syphilis.
    D. herpes simplex virus type 2.

❖ Critical Thinking ❖
Case Study

Bryan, age 14, has come to the clinic because he has started breaking out on his face, chest, and shoulders with acne. He says he is embarrassed to go out because his friends stare at him and girls avoid him. The physician has started medical treatment and sent him to you for further guidance.

29. Based on the above information, a priority nursing diagnosis for Bryan at this time would be:
    A. altered family processes related to the adolescent with a skin problem.
    B. body image disturbance related to perception of acne lesions.
    C. bathing/hygiene self-care deficit related to skin care.
    D. altered role performance related to perceived peer separation.

30. The BEST goal for Bryan would be which of the following?
    A. will have a positive body image
    B. will receive appropriate education for hygiene
    C. will have a reduction in dietary fat and calories
    D. will receive appropriate referral to skin specialist

31. Subjective data collection should include which of the following?
    A. family history of acne
    B. appropriate use of greasy cleansing creams, tars, and oils
    C. location and size description of visible lesions
    D. culture and sensitivity for identifying organism

32. The nurse has established a plan of care with Bryan. Which one of the following would be an expected component of the plan to improve Bryan's body image?

A. Help adolescent find mechanisms to reduce emotional stress.

B. Explain the disorder and therapy prescribed to increase family understanding.

C. Emphasize the positive aspects, as well as limited nature of the disorder, and assist with grooming to enhance appearance.

D. Discourage peer relationships until the adolescent has improved facial appearance from medication.

❖ Crossword Puzzle ❖

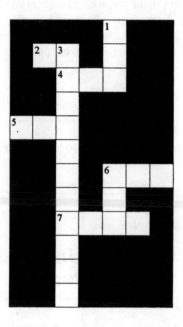

Across

2. Infectious mononucleosis
4. Intrauterine device
5. Centers for Disease Control
6. Pregnancy-induced hypertension
7. Intravenous drug user

Down

1. Sexually transmitted disease
3. Spontaneous abortion
6. Pelvic inflammatory disease

❖ CHAPTER 21
Behavioral Health Problems of Adolescence

1. Identify the following statements as either TRUE or FALSE.

_____ The number of fat cells may be established at an early age, and overfeeding during this time may have a significant influence on the development of obesity at a later age.

_____ Obesity is the most common nutritional disturbance of children.

_____ During the adolescent growth spurt, the distribution of fat in girls decreases sharply.

_____ Obesity refers to the state of weighing more than average for height and body build and may or may not include an increased amount of fat.

_____ Birth weight is an indicator of childhood obesity.

_____ In Prader-Willi syndrome, children manifest slow intellectual development, short stature, and obesity and will go to great lengths to obtain food.

_____ Obesity in adolescents can be caused by overeating or low activity levels.

_____ Obese persons eat more at a given sitting and tend to eat more rapidly than those who are not obese.

_____ Obese adolescents are characteristically night eaters and skip meals, especially breakfast.

_____ Obese children are often the product of families in which large meals are emphasized or children are scolded for leaving food on their plates.

2. Gail, age 14, comes to the school nurse's office because she is obese and wants to lose weight. The nurse's assessment will include:
A. Gail's physical activity.
B. dietary intake and meal patterns for Gail.
C. eating patterns of Gail's family.
D. all of the above.

3. Adolescents with obesity have common emotional problems of:
A. poor body image.
B. low self-esteem.
C. social isolation and feelings of rejection.
D. all of the above.

4. List three factors that can contribute to the development of a disturbed body image in the obese adolescent.

_____

_____

_____

5. The method of body composition measurement recommended for use with adolescents is:
   A. measurement of skinfold thickness.
   B. body mass index.
   C. bioelectric impedance.
   D. computed tomography.

6. Weight reduction management in adolescents should include:
   A. significant caloric restriction.
   B. elimination of physical hunger cues.
   C. regular physical activity.
   D. appetite-suppressant drugs.

7. The onset of anorexia nervosa has two peaks, between _____ years of age and between

   _____ years of age. This disorder is characterized by _____.

8. Individuals with bulimia are classified into two categories: those that _____

   and those that _____.

9. Cindy, age 16, has been sent to the school nurse because her gym teacher has noticed a marked decrease in Cindy's
   weight since vacation. Which one of the following does the nurse recognize as a common finding among adolescent
   girls with anorexia nervosa?
   A. wears form-fitting clothes like tank tops and jeans
   B. has strong peer relationships with classmates and several best friends
   C. has poor schoolwork performance because of little interest in school
   D. is present at meals, selects foods, and appears to family and friends to be eating appropriately

10. Cindy has been diagnosed with anorexia nervosa. Her therapeutic management plan includes hospitalization. Which
    one of the following would the nurse recognize as a possible reaction to the treatment plan?
    A. high energy level activity participation, especially with marked preoccupation with food preparation
    B. becoming dependent on her parents, especially her mother
    C. attempts to control the situation and views the treatment plan as an attempt to remove her autonomy
    D. regards her appearance as abnormal or ugly

11. Cindy is about to be discharged post treatment for anorexia nervosa. The nurse has formulated a nursing diagnosis
    related to family coping with a goal that the family will be prepared for home care. Which one of the following inter-
    ventions would BEST help meet this goal?
    A. Make certain both patient and family understand the therapeutic plan.
    B. Observe family interaction for assessment of family coping patterns.
    C. Explore feelings and attitudes of family members.
    D. Convey an attitude of caring and acceptance to family and patient.

12. Bulimia is observed most frequently in _____. _____
    bulimics are uncommon.

13. Karen is suspected of being bulimic. The nurse recognizes which of the following as clinical manifestations of this
    disease?
    A. often starts with inappropriate dietary intake because of the dissatisfaction felt from obesity in an effort to increase
       satisfaction, lower weight, and lower guilt feelings
    B. Once started, the binges decrease in frequency to only about seven to eight times per day.
    C. may have a caloric intake of 20,000 to 30,000 calories per day
    D. Insulin production is decreased because of excessive self-induced vomiting.

14. The patient with bulimia must be watched by the nurse for medical complications. Which one of the following does the nurse recognize as needing immediate intervention?
    A. backs of the hands scarred and cut from self-induced vomiting
    B. potassium depletion from diuretic abuse
    C. erosion of teeth enamel from self-induced vomiting
    D. chronic esophagitis from self-induced vomiting

15. Identify the following statements about substance abuse as either TRUE or FALSE.

    _____ A person may be physically dependent on a narcotic without being addicted.

    _____ The adolescent abusing drugs has often adopted the use of a substance as a means of coping with feelings of depression, boredom, and emptiness.

    _____ Identification of the pattern of drug use in the adolescent is essential but offers little help in developing a successful approach to the problem.

    _____ The usual goal for the compulsive drug user is one of peer acceptance.

    _____ One of the hazards associated with drug use is the risk of injury while driving under the influence of the drug.

16. Which one of the following adolescents does the nurse recognize as LEAST likely to begin smoking?
    A. Johnny, age 16, whose dad quit smoking two years ago
    B. Karen, age 13, whose older sister smokes
    C. Ted, age 17, who smokes a cigarette at home in front of his parents
    D. Robert, age 17, who comes from a low socioeconomic level and who does not participate in school activities

17. Johnny, age 16, has tried his first cigarette because of peer pressure to "look cool." What stage of becoming a smoker might the nurse label Johnny?
    A. preparation
    B. initiation
    C. experimentation
    D. regular smoking

18. The school nurse is planning an educational program centered on smoking prevention for junior high school adolescents. Which of the following methods does the nurse recognize as the MOST effective way to present this program?
    A. Ban smoking in the school.
    B. Teach methods of resistance to peer pressure for smoking.
    C. Use peer-led programs that emphasize social consequences of smoking.
    D. Use media videotapes and films dealing with smoking prevention.

19. Adolescent alcoholics are often described as:
    A. hard to live with and indecisive.
    B. good students with a strong desire to complete school.
    C. rarely denying their problem.
    D. having poor role models but excellent peer relations.

20. The motivation phase of treatment and rehabilitation of young drug users is directed toward:
    A. assessment of the drug habits and amount of drugs used.
    B. exploring the factors that influence drug use.
    C. prevention of relapse into drug use.
    D. all of the above.

21. The increase in suicide and depression during adolescence may be due to:
    A. expected low self-esteem among this population.
    B. the importance of peer pressures among this group.
    C. cognitive development and self-observation development among this group.
    D. higher substance abuse among this group.

22. Jim, who has no history of previous suicide attempt, is talking with the school nurse about his feelings of despair and hopelessness about the future. He tells the nurse he would be better off dead. The nurse's BEST response is which of the following?
    A. Recognize that Jim is going through a common phase of adolescence.
    B. Recognize that Jim is at low risk for suicide since he has not previously attempted suicide.
    C. Explain to Jim that suicide never solved anything and that he will feel better tomorrow.
    D. Take Jim seriously, allow time for him to verbalize his feelings, and stay with him until referral.

23. The nurse has been asked to present an educational program on prevention of adolescent stress and suicide. In planning the program, the nurse should include:
    A. the importance of being supportive and establishing positive communication patterns between family and teens.
    B. the precipitating factors for suicide.
    C. effective coping mechanisms and problem-solving skills.
    D. all of the above.

❖ Critical Thinking ❖
Case Study

Kenny, 16 years old, visits the clinic for follow-up of a recent infection. While talking with the nurse, he tells her that he has recently broken up with his girlfriend after going steady for 11 months. Kenny has a history of having a difficult home situation. His recent school performance has declined, and this has further upset Kenny's parents and their expectations for him. Physical examination of Kenny reveals an expressionless face with a slight smell of alcohol on his breath and signs consistent with depression.

24. You suspect that Kenny might be suicidal. Which factors in the above data might support this assumption?
    1. alcohol consumption
    2. recent breakup with girlfriend
    3. history of difficult home situation
    4. depression
    5. age and gender
    A. 1, 2, 3, and 4
    B. 2, 3, and 4
    C. 2, 4, and 5
    D. 1, 2, 3, 4, and 5

25. Upon questioning by the nurse, Kenny admits to suicidal ideation. What should the nurse first assess to determine risk?
    A. history of suicide attempts within the family
    B. past methods of coping with stress by the individual
    C. whether Kenny has a plan for suicide
    D. whether Kenny has a gun available

26. Which one of the following nursing diagnoses would the nurse develop to BEST deal with Kenny's suicide thoughts?
    A. high risk for injury related to feelings of rejection
    B. sleep pattern disturbance related to inability to sleep
    C. social isolation related to withdrawal from friends
    D. high risk for self-directed violence related to excessive alcohol use

27. The MOST important goal in the nursing management of Kenny at this time should focus on:
    A. reestablishing Kenny's relationship with his girlfriend.
    B. teaching Kenny how to cope with the stress of being an adolescent.
    C. maintaining physical safety for Kenny.
    D. assisting Kenny to express his emotional pain and regain his ability to perform assigned tasks.

❖ Crossword Puzzle ❖

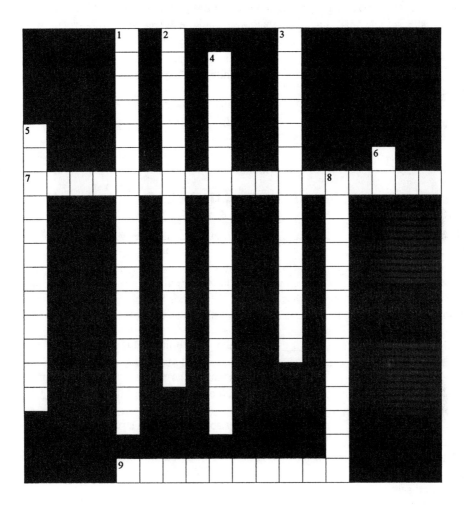

Across

7. An adaptive physiologic state that occurs when a drug is taken in increasing amounts (2 words)
9. The overzealous use of drugs or the exercise of bad judgment in their use (2 words)

Down

1. Overwhelming involvement with obtaining and using a narcotic for its psychic effects (2 words)
2. An act made without any real attempt to cause serious injury or death (2 words)
3. An act intended to cause self-injury or death (2 words)
4. Thoughts about or plans for suicide (2 words)
5. A rage response designed to punish or manipulate a loved person (2 words)
6. Anorexia nervosa
8. The clinical need to increase the dosage of a drug in order to attain the same effect (2 words)

❖ CHAPTER 22
Family-Centered Care of the Child with Chronic Illness or Disability

1. Match the term with its definition.

   A. chronic illness

   B. congenital disability

   C. developmental delay

   D. developmental disability

   E. disability

   F. handicap

   G. impairment

   H. technology-dependent child

   I. home care

   J. normalization

   K. mainstreaming

   _____ a barrier imposed by society

   _____ principle that permits disabled children to remain a part of their community

   _____ a child that requires the routine use of a medical device for support of a bodily function

   _____ a condition that interferes with daily functioning for more than three months

   _____ functional limitation

   _____ a system of care that minimizes the disruptive impact of the child's condition on the family

   _____ a maturational lag

   _____ a disability that has existed since birth

   _____ any lifelong disability that is manifested before age 22 years

   _____ process that has largely resulted from the passage of Public Law 94-142, the Education for All Handicapped Children Act of 1975

   _____ a loss or abnormality of a structure or function

2. Which one of the following diseases is listed among both the most lethal and the most common diseases?
   A. asthma
   B. congenital heart disease
   C. cancer
   D. spina bifida

3. Which of the following chronic illnesses have had markedly improved survival rates in recent years?
   1. Hodgkin disease and leukemia
   2. cystic fibrosis and spina bifida
   3. asthma and muscular dystrophy
   4. preterm and low-birth-weight infants
   A. 4 only
   B. 1 and 2
   C. 1, 2, and 4
   D. 2, 3, and 4

4. A goal that would be considered INAPPROPRIATE for family-centered care would be to:
   A. maintain the integrity of the family.
   B. empower the family members.
   C. support the family during stressful times.
   D. maintain a high level of control.

Fill in the blanks in the following statements.

5. _____ _____ _____ parents usually have a high level of trust in the nurse with a low-level need for information.

6. Parents who fit in the _____ _____ category do not initiate relationships with nurses and are difficult to engage in decision making.

7. If the parent is in control of health-related decisions and uses the nurses for consultation and direct care, he/she can be said to follow the pattern of _____ _____ _____.

8. Parents who keep track of the staff and seek detailed information would be referred to as _____

   _____ _____.

9. Nurses who use a _____ approach try to remove barriers to parents' participation.

10. A nurse who tends to need a high degree of control over his/her work may take the role of _____

    _____ with parents.

11. When conflict arises with the level of trust the parents have in the professional, the problem is usually:
    A. from the fact that most nurses use a "rule enforcer" approach to interaction.
    B. one that could have been avoided if the nurse had used an individualized approach to interaction.
    C. that the parents use a manager of care approach to their interaction.
    D. the family members were empowered and made an inadvisable choice.

12. The Individual Family Service Plan (IFSP) is:
    A. developed jointly by families and professionals.
    B. a comprehensive insurance plan for families with a disabled child.
    C. developed by a team of professionals for the disabled child.
    D. contained in strategies for the school-age disabled child.

13. When working with people of other cultural backgrounds, nurses should place an emphasis on:
    A. promoting independent living.
    B. requiring family participation.
    C. viewing their child as disabled.
    D. planning to meet the family's needs.

14. If the reaction of a family member to the diagnosis of a chronic illness is denial, the nurse would recognize that denial is:
    A. an abnormal response to grieving this type of loss.
    B. preventing treatment and rehabilitation.
    C. necessary to prevent a crisis.
    D. necessary for the child's optimum development.

15. Health professionals work with people in denial frequently, but many health professionals typically do NOT:
    A. actively attempt to remove the denial behaviors.
    B. repeatedly give blunt explanations.
    C. label denial as maladaptive.
    D. understand the concept of denial.

16. Hope in the terminally ill child's family would be considered:
    A. a way to absorb stress in a manageable way.
    B. negative coping with a serious diagnosis.
    C. a maladaptive mechanism for dealing with the inevitable death.
    D. to have the same meaning for the nurse and the family.

17. The BEST sign that a young child has fully adjusted to his/her terminal illness is that he/she:
    A. believes that procedures are inflicted as a punishment.
    B. talks about the disease and its effect on his/her life.
    C. passively accepts painful procedures.
    D. expresses anger about the restrictions imposed by the disease.

18. Which of the following types of parental reactions to the child with a chronic illness is characterized by parents who detach themselves emotionally but provide adequate physical care?
    A. overprotection
    B. denial
    C. gradual acceptance
    D. rejection

19. List at least five characteristics of parental overprotection.

    _____

    _____

    _____

    _____

    _____

20. When the parents of a child with special needs experience chronic sorrow, the process:
    A. of grief is pronounced and self-limiting.
    B. involves social reintegration after grieving.
    C. is characterized by realistic expectations.
    D. is interspersed with periods of intensified grief.

21. Placement of a disabled child out of the home usually occurs if the:
    A. child has been successfully maintained within the home.
    B. child's needs are progressively met.
    C. integrity of the family unit is in jeopardy.
    D. family is maladjusted.

22. Which one of the following stressors can usually be anticipated in a child with special needs?
    A. the approximate cost of the yearly medical bills
    B. the future needs for residential care
    C. the types of schooling and vocational training that will be needed
    D. the developmental milestones and the start of school causing stress of some kind

23. If the parent is interacting with the disabled child in an unrewarding and minimally productive way, the nurse might recommend for the parent:
    A. education about reasonable expectations.
    B. assistance to identify the child's strengths.
    C. to enroll the child in respite care.
    D. all of the above.

24. One sign that parents are NOT using a shared approach to the care of the child with a chronic illness is:
    A. when the father does not provide any physical care.
    B. tasks are divided in a very specific way.
    C. one parent is absent from the hospital.
    D. marital conflict.

25. Which one of the following factors is more characteristic of a father's pattern than a mother's pattern of adjusting to a chronically ill child? The father is more likely to:
    A. feel a threat to his self-esteem.
    B. report a periodic crisis pattern.
    C. forfeit personal goals.
    D. seek immediate professional counseling.

26. Which one of the following statements is FALSE about marital relationships of parents with a disabled child?
    A. Conflicts in parental roles place a strain on the relationship.
    B. Most families manage the strain.
    C. Divorce rates are higher than those for the general population.
    D. The best predictor of long-term marital adjustment is the couple's previous marital functioning.

27. Define *courtesy stigma*.

    _____

    _____

28. Which one of the following characteristics would be considered abnormal in a sibling relationship?
    A. sharing
    B. withdrawal
    C. competing
    D. compromising

29. Society's negative views of disabled children are often a result of:
    A. ignorance and limited resources.
    B. ignorance and fear.
    C. the unpredictable nature of the disorders.
    D. ambivalence and fear.

30. The level of adjustment that families with a disabled child experience is MOST significantly influenced by the:
    A. functional burden.
    B. severity of the condition.
    C. family's perception of the condition.
    D. available resources.

31. The effectiveness of the available support system depends upon the:
    A. sources of the support and their availability.
    B. sources of the support and their communication.
    C. extended family and their availability.
    D. extended family and their resources.

32. Which one of the following statements is FALSE about family members' perceptions of the child's illness or disability?
   A. Children may interpret the reason for the illness/disability as a punishment.
   B. Family members are usually shocked to learn that their child has a serious illness/disability.
   C. Parents may interpret illness/disability as a punishment.
   D. Family members usually have no knowledge about the disorder when they learn their child has it.

33. Identify each of the following coping behaviors as either an *approach* behavior or an *avoidance* behavior.

   _____ A. A father stops at a friend's house and talks about his child's poor prognosis.

   _____ B. A father's alcohol use increases to the point of being excessive.

   _____ C. A father calls to ask his insurance agent about health insurance coverage after the child reaches 18 years of age.

   _____ D. A mother tells the nurse that she is afraid to tell her child about his/her poor prognosis.

   _____ E. A mother does not carry a glucose source for her toddler who takes insulin for type I diabetes mellitus.

   _____ F. A mother begins to cry in the nurse's office at school, saying that she always gets depressed at the beginning of the new year.

   _____ G. A father explains how the hemodialysis machine works.

   _____ H. A father asks the nurse to explain the diagnosis again.

   _____ I. A mother uses herbs instead of the prescribed inhaler to treat her child's asthma episode.

   _____ J. A mother asks her neighbor to watch her older child for a few hours while she is at the clinic.

34. Match the developmental stage with the particular challenge/risk that a disability would usually impart at this age.

   A. infant   _____ self-image

   B. toddler   _____ social development

   C. preschooler   _____ attachment

   D. school-age child _____ mobility

   E. adolescent   _____ participation

35. Which one of the following coping mechanisms is more characteristic of a well child than a disabled child?
   A. develops competence
   B. submission or endurance
   C. complies with treatment
   D. seeks support

36. The disabled child tends to develop appropriate independence and achievement when the parents:
   A. protect the child from all dangers.
   B. establish reasonable limits.
   C. emphasize their limits.
   D. isolate the child to avoid peer rejection.

37. Which one of the following factors places the disabled child at greatest risk for ineffective coping?
   A. a severe disorder
   B. a physical disability
   C. multiple conditions
   D. inability to think abstractly

38. The purpose of the initial assessment of the disabled child's coping mechanisms is for the nurse to:
   A. identify strengths and reactions to the disorder.
   B. establish a rapport with the child and family.
   C. provide care from stage to stage of development.
   D. provide care from phase to phase of the disorder.

39. Which of the following statements about the time of diagnosis is FALSE?
   A. Parents may not remember all that is said.
   B. Parents remember the tone of the communication.
   C. Parents cannot sense the tone of communication.
   D. Parents may not hear all that is said.

40. The primary purpose for including both parents in the initial informing interview is to:
   A. observe the interaction between the parents.
   B. provide mutual support.
   C. avoid marital conflict.
   D. permit expression of their emotions.

41. List the three most common family responses to the diagnosis of a chronic illness or disability.

   _____

   _____

   _____

42. Which of the following is the MOST effective method of support to the family who is responding with denial to a diagnosis of a chronic disorder or disability?
   A. use of body language
   B. listening
   C. concentration
   D. all of the above

43. Which of the following strategies is INAPPROPRIATE when dealing with a parent who is experiencing feelings of guilt about his/her child's diagnosis of a chronic disorder or disability?
   A. Encourage the parent to express his/her feelings.
   B. Explain in detail the causes of the disorder.
   C. Acknowledge the parent's feelings.
   D. Encourage the irrationality of the thought.

44. The nurse should respond to anger in parents of the disabled child with:
    A. reciprocal anger.
    B. disapproval.
    C. acceptance.
    D. avoidance.

45. Corbin and Strauss's "chronic illness trajectory" model is based on the idea that the:
    A. family understands the meaning of the illness situation.
    B. course of the illness changes over time.
    C. family member roles change with illness.
    D. coping patterns for the illness can be learned.

46. Nurses who provide support to parents of a child with a disability should develop an attitude that has all of the following characteristics EXCEPT the belief that:
    A. every person has burdens to bear.
    B. trust is a foundation for good communication.
    C. parents are experts about their own child.
    D. parents are equal to professionals.

47. The father of a disabled child is often:
    A. directly involved in the provision of care.
    B. socialized to express his concerns.
    C. without adequate emotional support.
    D. directly involved in the medical decision making.

48. The adaptive coping process includes:
    A. cognitive tasks.
    B. behavioral tasks.
    C. emotional tasks.
    D. all of the above.

49. The Crippled Children's Services, which provides financial assistance for children with many disabling conditions, is now known as:
    A. Programs for Children with Special Health Needs.
    B. National Information Center for Children and Youth With Disabilities.
    C. Association for the Care of Children's Health.
    D. Alliance for Health, Physical Education, Recreation and Dance.

50. When identifying parents to offer support to other parents of disabled children, the selected individuals should have all of the following requirements EXCEPT:
    A. advocacy and problem-solving skills.
    B. a child with the same diagnosis.
    C. nonjudgmental approach to problem solving.
    D. good listening skills.

❖ Critical Thinking ❖
Case Study

Jerome Thomas is a 15-month-old who was born prematurely and was discharged from the hospital at age 3 months after multiple invasive procedures, intubation, ventilation, and surgery. He is delayed in his motor development, but other areas of development are progressing as would be expected for a prematurely born infant of his age. Jerome has recently been labeled as having cerebral palsy. He is at the physician's office for a routine health check. His mother is with him.

51. In order to assess the family's adjustment to the diagnosis, the nurse would gather more information. One area that could be deferred to a later date would be the assessment of his:
    A. developmental level.
    B. available support system.
    C. family's coping mechanisms.
    D. family's goals for the future.

Jerome's mother has returned to work part-time as a partner in a computer consulting firm. Jerome's father is a marketing consultant in the food industry and travels a lot. The couple has hired a woman who comes into the home whom they trust with Jerome's many needs. Jerome goes out of the home several times a week for therapy. Jerome is an only child. His parents are in their late thirties.

52. Based on the information given above, what is the BEST nursing diagnosis for Jerome?
    A. high risk for injury
    B. altered family processes
    C. altered growth and development
    D. impaired social interaction

53. With the selected diagnosis in mind, what is the expected outcome with the highest priority for Jerome?
    A. Jerome will achieve physical development of a 15-month-old.
    B. Jerome will achieve psychosocial and cognitive development of a 15-month-old.
    C. Jerome's parents express both positive and negative reactions to Jerome's progress.
    D. Jerome's parents will set realistic goals for themselves and Jerome.

54. Which one of the following interventions would be appropriate for Jerome's parents to begin at this time?
    A. Institute age-appropriate limit-setting.
    B. Encourage mastery of self-help skills.
    C. Help Jerome deal with criticism.
    D. Help Jerome realize that his disability is not a punishment.

55. Between now and Jerome's next visit at 24 months, the nurse should teach the parents that developmentally, Jerome will be developing:
    A. a sense of trust and attachment to his parents.
    B. mastery of self-care skills.
    C. a sense of body image.
    D. through sensorimotor experiences.

❖ Crossword Puzzle ❖

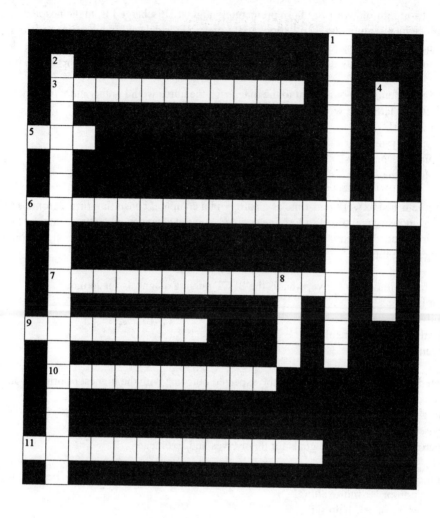

Across

3. Means by which families acquire a sense of control over their family lives
5. Individual Education Program
6. Coping behaviors that result in movement toward adjustment and resolution of a crisis (2 words)
7. Establishing a normal pattern of living
9. An environmental barrier that prevents or makes difficult full integration
10. The restriction or lack of ability to perform normally as a result of impairment
11. The integration of special-needs children into regular classrooms

Down

1. A condition that interferes with daily functioning for more than three months in a year or causes hospitalization of more than one month in a year (2 words)
2. A maturational lag (2 words)
4. A loss or abnormality of structure or function
8. Individual Family Service Plan

❖ CHAPTER 23
Family-Centered Care of the Child with Life-Threatening Illness

1. Which one of the following diseases has increased in incidence in all age groups of children in the years from 1985 to 1990?
   A. acquired immunodeficiency syndrome (AIDS)
   B. cancer
   C. injuries
   D. malignant neoplasms

2. Which one of the following techniques would be considered an example of the MOST therapeutic communication to use with the bereaved family?
   A. cheerfulness
   B. interpretation
   C. validating loss
   D. reassurance

3. Which one of the following helping statements would be LEAST therapeutic for the nurse to use with the bereaved family?
   A. "You can stay with him and hold him if you wish."
   B. "It must be painful for you to return to the doctor's office without her."
   C. "Fortunately, his suffering is over now."
   D. "Will your husband return to be with you soon?"

4. Which one of the following age groups will be MOST likely to suffer negative reactions to an altered body image as the result of a life-threatening illness?
   A. toddlers
   B. school-age children
   C. adolescents
   D. All age groups are affected equally.

5. List at least five reasons that a nurse becomes an important part of the therapeutic team when the child has a life-threatening disease.

   _____

   _____

   _____

   _____

6. Parents of a child in remission from cancer who is being discharged are advised to:
   A. schedule return appointments to give the child a break in the routine.
   B. resume rules and limits that were in effect before the illness.
   C. increase vigilance and liberalize the discipline.
   D. indulge the child while they can.

7. Which of the following strategies would enhance compliance in adolescents?
   A. Include the adolescent in the treatment discussions.
   B. Help the family set clear expectations.
   C. Clarify roles and provide written instructions.
   D. all of the above

8. Because many children with cancer are treated in tertiary centers, they will:
   A. have one primary nurse to act as liaison.
   B. be ensured continuity of care.
   C. often lack preventive interventions.
   D. be only a short distance from home.

9. At the time therapy is terminated, many parents:
   A. express ambivalence.
   B. readily give up the medical regimen.
   C. have a psychologic need for the child's sick role.
   D. need less support than at the time of diagnosis.

10. A family's reaction during the terminal stage of illness involves a period of intense anticipatory grieving characterized by:
    A. depression.
    B. loss of hope.
    C. intensification of fears.
    D. all of the above.

11. When the parent of a child who is dying tells the nurse the child is in pain even when the child appears comfortable, the nurse should be sure that:
    A. p.r.n. pain control measures are instituted.
    B. pain control is administered on a preventive schedule.
    C. parents understand that pain is a physical process.
    D. parents understand that the child is probably in less pain than he/she appears.

12. List at least five physical signs of approaching death.

    _____

    _____

    _____

    _____

    _____

13. Which one of the following interventions is MOST important for the dying child?
    A. emotional support
    B. preparing parents to deal with fears
    C. relief from pain
    D. control of pain

14. Which one of the following strategies would be BEST for the nurse to use to support the family's spiritual needs when their child's death is imminent?
    A. Pray with the family.
    B. Implement relaxation techniques.
    C. Make an appointment for the family to speak with an expert.
    D. all of the above

15. The extended phase of mourning:
    A. usually takes about a year.
    B. is accompanied by support of the family at the funeral.
    C. may extend over years.
    D. can be eliminated if the family is well prepared.

16. When a child dies suddenly, which one of the following interventions would be LEAST beneficial?
    A. Avoid having the family view the body of a disfigured child.
    B. Inform the family of what to expect when they see the disfigured body of their child.
    C. Offer the parents the opportunity to see the child's body even after resuscitation was performed.
    D. Arrange to have a health care worker with bereavement training remain with the family.

17. Match the cognitive stage with the child's concept of death at that stage.

    A. sensorimotor   _____ Death is irreversible, universal, and inevitable, with physiologic and theo-
                                        logic explanations.

    B. preoperational
                               _____ Death is temporary and reversible.

    C. concrete operations
                               _____ Death is irreversible, with physiologic and naturalistic explanations, but not
    D. formal operations   necessarily inevitable.

                               _____ There is no concept of death, but child reacts to loss.

18. Fear of the unknown is one of the greatest threats to seriously ill children of which age group?
    A. toddlers
    B. preschoolers
    C. school-age children
    D. adolescents

19. Immobilization is one of the greatest threats to seriously ill children of which age group?
    A. toddlers
    B. preschoolers
    C. school-age children
    D. adolescents

20. Fear of punishment is one of the greatest threats to seriously ill children of which age group?
    A. toddlers
    B. preschoolers
    C. school-age children
    D. adolescents

21. Inability to use their parents for emotional support is one of the greatest threats to seriously ill children of which age group?
    A. toddlers
    B. preschoolers
    C. school-age children
    D. adolescents

22. When assisting parents to support their dying child, the nurse should stress the importance of honesty, because if parents are honest and openly discuss their fears the child is more likely to:
    A. discuss his/her fears.
    B. ask fewer distressing questions.
    C. lose his/her sense of hope.
    D. all of the above

23. The sibling of a dying child may feel:
    A. left out and unimportant.
    B. concern for his/her own health.
    C. physical symptoms similar to his/her sibling's.
    D. all of the above.

24. The nurse should recommend to the parents of a child who is dying that the sibling usually needs to:
    A. be protected from the reasons for the death.
    B. receive information about what is happening.
    C. be observed for the abnormal signs of anger or jealously.
    D. be excused from any of the care or chores related to the sick child.

25. Which of the following symptoms would be considered normal grief behavior?
    A. feeling the need to have friends and relatives around
    B. feeling an emotional closeness to friends and relatives
    C. hearing the dead person's voice
    D. all of the above

26. The process of mourning is usually completed:
    A. in sequential phases.
    B. in about two years.
    C. in about three years.
    D. in phases not related to time.

❖ Critical Thinking ❖
Case Study

Julie Casswell is a 6-year-old child with leukemia. She has undergone a bone marrow transplant with associated complications and has had several remissions. After the last remission she deteriorated rapidly and is now in the final stages of her illness. Her parents tell you that they are discouraged and depressed.

27. How should the nurse approach the parents in regard to their feelings about Julie's impending death?
    A. The nurse should begin with an assessment.
    B. The nurse should be sure that Julie's parents know that repeated relapses with remissions are associated with a better prognosis.
    C. The nurse should begin to help the parents work through their depression.
    D. The nurse should use heavy sedation to help Julie and her parents cope with this phase.

28. As Julie's parents express their concerns, it becomes very clear that pain control is a fear for Julie and her parents. What strategy should the nurse use to help them deal with this fear?
    A. The nurse should assure the parents that Julie's pain will be relieved.
    B. The nurse should use heavy sedation to help Julie and her parents cope with this phase.
    C. A medication schedule should be adopted that will prevent the pain from escalating.
    D. The pain medications should be given only intravenously when Julie is near death.

29. After Julie's death at Christmas time, which one of the following evaluation strategies is MOST likely to also help support and guide the family through the resolution of their loss?
    A. a written questionnaire
    B. a telephone call placed in early January
    C. a meeting with the family at time of death
    D. a telephone call placed in early February

30. Which one of the following choices would be the BEST choice of expected outcomes for the nursing diagnosis of fear/anxiety when planning care for Julie in this terminal stage?
   A. Julie will discuss her fears without evidence of stress.
   B. Julie will exhibit no evidence of loneliness.
   C. Julie's parents are actively involved in Julie's care.
   D. Julie's parents demonstrate ability to provide care for her.

❖ Crossword Puzzle ❖

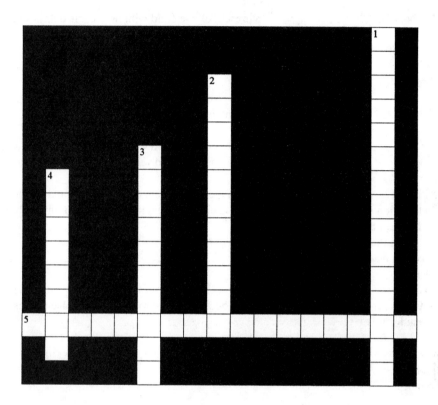

Across

5. Grieving before an actual loss (2 words)

Down

1. Condition wherein a life is near or approaching its end (2 words)
2. Period of mourning
3. Somatic symptoms and intense subjective distress that occur soon after a significant loss (2 words)
4. Prolonged process of resolving grief

❖ CHAPTER 24
The Child with Cognitive, Sensory, or Communication Impairment

1. Match the level of mental retardation/IQ range with the appropriate example of a child's maturation and/or development.

A. mild (50-55 to about 70)

_____ a preschool-age child with noticeable delays in motor development and in speech

B. moderate (35-40 to 50-55)

_____ an adult who may walk but who needs complete custodial care

C. severe (20-25 to 35-40)

_____ a school-age child who is able to walk and who can profit from systematic habit training

D. profound (below 20-25)

_____ a preschool-age child who may not be noticed as retarded but who is slow to walk, feed self, and talk

2. The classic definition of *mental retardation* differs from the more recent definition adopted by the American Association on Mental Retardation in that the new upper limit of subaverage intellectual functioning includes:
   A. an intelligence quotient that is lower.
   B. adaptive limitation in the criteria.
   C. only intelligence and no other criteria.
   D. an age limit of 12.

3. When teaching a child with a cognitive impairment, the BEST strategy for the nurse to use to present symbols in an exaggerated concrete form is:
   A. music.
   B. memorizing.
   C. verbal explanation.
   D. ignoring the child.

4. Define the term *fading*.

_____

_____

5. Define the term *shaping*.

_____

_____

6. Acquiring social skills for the cognitively impaired child includes:
   A. teaching acceptable sexual behavior.
   B. exposing the child to strangers.
   C. greeting visitors without being overly friendly.
   D. all of the above.

7. The percentage of cognitively impaired adolescents who have had sexual intercourse is:
   A. less than the general population.
   B. greater than the general population.
   C. about the same as the general population.
   D. near zero.

8. The reasons that parents often give for seeking sterilization for their mentally retarded child include:
   A. contraception.
   B. to eliminate menses.
   C. to avoid hygiene problems.
   D. all of the above.

9. The BEST contraceptive choice for the cognitively impaired child that would require little compliance, produce amenorrhea, and provide long-term protection from pregnancy is:
   A. the intrauterine device.
   B. levonorgestrel implant (Norplant).
   C. hysterectomy.
   D. oral contraception.

10. Define *task analysis* and describe its use when teaching a mentally retarded child.

_____

_____

_____

_____

11. The primary purpose of recordkeeping for seven days prior to toilet training a mentally retarded child is to:
    A. determine patterns of behavior and parents' response.
    B. determine the amount of urinary output.
    C. determine the parents' willingness to participate.
    D. All of the above are equally important.

12. The mutual participation model of care for the cognitively impaired child who needs hospitalization would include:
    A. isolating the child from others to avoid conflicts.
    B. encouraging the parents to room in.
    C. having the parents perform all of the activities of daily living.
    D. having the nurse perform all of the activities of daily living.

13. Another name for trisomy 21 is:
    A. phenylketonuria.
    B. Turner syndrome.
    C. Down syndrome.
    D. galactosemia.

14. Genetic counseling for parents of a child with Down syndrome is:
    A. necessary whenever there is mosaicism.
    B. necessary whenever there is translocation.
    C. always necessary.
    D. seldom necessary.

15. According to Carr and Cooper, families who keep the Down syndrome child at home report having:
    A. more negative feelings for the child.
    B. a more accepting attitude toward others.
    C. higher divorce rates.
    D. more sibling problems.

16. Fragile X syndrome is:
    A. the most common inherited cause of mental retardation.
    B. the most common inherited cause of mental retardation next to Down syndrome.
    C. caused by an abnormal gene on chromosome 21.
    D. caused by a missing gene on the X chromosome.

17. Genetic counseling for parents of a child with fragile X syndrome is:
    A. necessary whenever there is permutation.
    B. necessary whenever there is translocation.
    C. always necessary.
    D. seldom necessary.

18. The correct term to use for a person whose hearing disability precludes successful processing of linguistic information through audition is:
    A. deaf-mute.
    B. mute.
    C. deaf.
    D. deaf and dumb.

19. Conductive hearing loss in children is most often a result of:
    A. use of tobramycin and gentamicin.
    B. high noise levels from ventilators.
    C. congenital defects.
    D. recurrent serous otitis media.

20. In the assessment of an infant to identify whether a hearing impairment has developed, the nurse would look for:
    A. a monotone voice.
    B. consistent lack of the startle reflex.
    C. a louder than usual cry.
    D. inability to form the word "da da" by 6 months.

21. In the assessment of a child to identify whether a hearing impairment has developed, the nurse would look for:
    A. a loud monotone voice.
    B. consistent lack of the startle reflex.
    C. a high level of social activity.
    D. attentiveness, especially when someone is talking.

22. All of the following are strategies that will enhance communication with a child who is hearing impaired EXCEPT:
    A. touch the child lightly to signal presence of a speaker.
    B. speak at eye level or a 45-degree angle.
    C. use facial expressions to convey message better.
    D. move and use animated body language to communicate better.

23. Match the type of visual impairment with its description.

A. myopia   _____   increased intraocular pressure

B. hyperopia   _____   squint or crossed eyes

C. astigmatism   _____   different refractive strength in each eye

D. anisometropia   _____   unequal curvatures in refractive apparatus

E. amblyopia   _____   opacity of crystalline lens

F. strabismus   _____   farsightedness

G. cataracts   _____   lazy eye

H. glaucoma   _____   nearsightedness

24. If a child has a penetrating injury to the eye, the nurse should:
    A. apply an eye patch.
    B. attempt to remove the object.
    C. irrigate the eye.
    D. use strict aseptic technique to examine the eye.

25. Which of the following situations would be considered abnormal?
    A. a newborn who does not consistently follow a bright toy with his eyes
    B. a toddler whose mother says she looks cross-eyed
    C. a 5-year-old who has hyperopia
    D. presence of a red reflex in a 7-year-old

26. Define the term *blindism*.

    _____

    _____

27. List at least eight of the strategies that the nurse can use during hospitalization with a child who has lost his/her sight.

    _____   _____

    _____   _____

    _____   _____

    _____   _____

28. Which of the following statements is CORRECT about eye care and sports?
    A. Glasses may interfere with the child's ability in sports.
    B. Face mask and helmet should be required gear for softball.
    C. Contact lenses provide less visual acuity than glasses for sports.
    D. It is usually very difficult to convince children to wear their glasses to play sports.

29. The method of communication used with the deaf-blind child that involves spelling into the child's hand is called:
    A. finger spelling.
    B. the Tadoma method.
    C. blindism.
    D. the tapping method.

30. Which one of the following examples would be MOST indicative of a language disorder?
    A. a 22-month-old child who has not uttered his first word
    B. a 36-month-old who has not formed his first sentence
    C. an 18-month-old who uses short "telegraphic" phrases
    D. a 4-year-old whose speech is not entirely understandable

31. Which of the following statements about stuttering is CORRECT?
    A. Stuttering is normal in the school-age child.
    B. Stuttering occurs because children do not know what they want to say.
    C. Undue emphasis on stuttering may cause an abnormal speech pattern.
    D. Chances for reversal of stuttering are good until about age 3.

32. The parents of a child who is stuttering should be encouraged to:
    A. have the child start again more slowly.
    B. give the child plenty of time.
    C. show concern for the hesitancy.
    D. reward the child for proper speech.

❖ Critical Thinking ❖
Case Study

Paula Larson is a 9-month-old infant with Down syndrome (DS) who is admitted to the hospital with pneumonia. She holds her head steady but cannot sit without support or pull up on the furniture. Paula squeals and laughs but does not imitate speech sounds or use any words such as "da da" or "ma ma." She can shake a rattle but cannot pass a block from one hand to the other. She smiles spontaneously and holds her own bottle, but she does not play "pattycake" or wave "bye bye."

Along with developmental deficits, Paula has several medical problems. She has congenital heart anomalies and is blind and deaf. She has been hospitalized many times for pneumonia and bronchiolitis.

Paula's parents knew that she would be born with DS. They have chosen to care for Paula at home. Paula's care has become increasingly more time-consuming; and during the admission assessment interview, Mr. and Mrs. Larson state they are both exhausted.

33. The nurse determines that Paula's developmental lag is LEAST pronounced in the area of:
    A. gross motor skills.
    B. language skills.
    C. fine motor skills.
    D. personal-social skills.

34. Paula's parents have cared for her at home since her birth. Mrs. Larson expresses concern that she is not doing a good enough job and that perhaps it is time to consider placement out of the home for Paula. The nurse responds based on the knowledge that the:
    A. potential for development varies greatly in DS.
    B. every available source of assistance to help the child and family should be explored.
    C. nurse's response may influence Mr. and Mrs. Larson's decisions.
    D. all of the above

35. Which one of the following common nursing diagnoses used in planning care for mentally retarded children should take priority in Paula's current situation?
    A. altered growth and development
    B. altered family processes
    C. anxiety related to hospitalization
    D. impaired social interaction

36. Mr. and Mrs. Larson make the decision to explore residential care for Paula. The BEST expected outcome during this time for Paula Larson would be for the parents to:
    A. demonstrate acceptance for Paula.
    B. express feelings and concerns regarding the implications of Paula's birth.
    C. make a realistic decision based on Paula's needs and capabilities as well as their own.
    D. identify realistic goals for Paula's future home care.

❖ Crossword Puzzle ❖

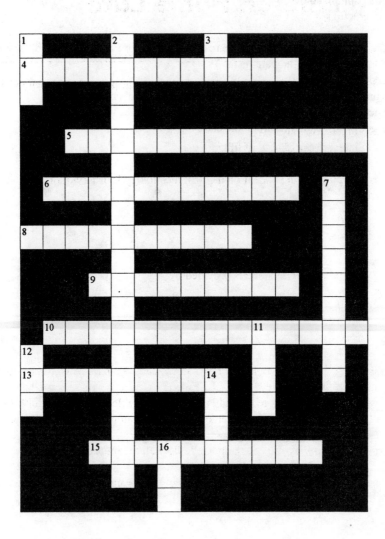

Across

4. Visual acuity between 20/70 and 20/200 (2 words)
5. Different reactive strength in each eye
6. Unequal curvatures in corneas or lenses
8. Understanding what is being said by watching movements of speaker's mouth and facial expressions (2 words)
9. Reduced visual acuity in one eye despite optical correction
10. Visual acuity of 20/200 or less (2 words)
13. Farsightedness
15. Absence of refractive errors

Down

1. American Sign Language
2. Mental deficiency (2 words)
3. Down syndrome
7. Self-stimulatory habits
11. Denver Articulation Screening Examination
12. Congenital heart disease
14. American Association on Mental Retardation
16. Educable mentally retarded

❖ CHAPTER 25
Family-Centered Home Care

1. The increase in the number of children who are cared for at home has probably been MOST influenced by:
   A. increased survival rates for children with leukemia.
   B. open heart surgery advances for congenital heart defects.
   C. advances in neonatal intensive care.
   D. consumer efforts to increase the quality of life.

2. The cost of home care for children dependent on medical technology is usually more than hospital care for:
   A. third-party payers.
   B. the government.
   C. the family.
   D. all of the above.

3. Some of the nursing care of children at home is provided by:
   A. registered nurses.
   B. home health aides.
   C. the family.
   D. all of the above.

4. Which one of the following situations would be of MOST concern to the nurse who is evaluating a family for the possibility of a discharge with home care?
   A. The preterm infant who will be managed with home care is unstable after surgery for his congenital heart anomaly.
   B. The family of a child who will be on total parenteral nutrition at home has no telephone.
   C. The parents are asking about the availability of respite care.
   D. The mother plans to stop working outside the home to be with the infant.

5. List the minimum contents of any written home care instructions for the child with complex home care requirements.

   _____

   _____

   _____

   _____

   _____

   _____

6. The BEST strategy to use when planning for transition from hospital to home for the child with complex home care requirements would be to:
   A. give the parents a trial period at home during which the parents provide some of the care.
   B. teach a family member all aspects of the child's care.
   C. allow the parents to provide total care in the hospital with support from the staff as needed.
   D. arrange a predischarge visit during the hospitalization by the home care nurse.

7. Ideally, home care of the child who is technology-dependent should be based on the concept of:
   A. traditional case management.
   B. independent care.
   C. primary care management.
   D. case management with care coordination.

8. According to the American Nurses Association, the qualifications of the nurse case manager should include:
   A. a baccalaureate degree in nursing.
   B. three years of experience.
   C. knowledge about community resources.
   D. all of the above.

9. The pediatric home care nurse's practice includes all of the following EXCEPT:
   A. consultation with peers to make most decisions.
   B. a high level of technical clinical expertise.
   C. knowledge of child development.
   D. the ability to support family autonomy.

10. List at least five aspects of care coordination in pediatric home care.

   _____

   _____

   _____

   _____

   _____

11. The pediatric nurse in home care practice would be expected to adhere to standards of practice developed by the:
    A. World Health Organization.
    B. American Nurses Association.
    C. Pediatric Nurses Society.
    D. National League for Nursing.

12. Strategies that promote the central goal of family-centered home care would include all of the following EXCEPT:
    A. emphasizing family strengths.
    B. identifying family coping mechanisms.
    C. identifying the family as dysfunctional.
    D. promoting family empowerment.

13. The LEARN framework for communication with families involves:

   L _____

   E _____

   A _____

   R _____

   N _____

14. Basic principles used to communicate with the family include all of the following EXCEPT:
    A. informing families who will have access to the information.
    B. assuring families that they have the right to confidentiality.
    C. collecting all information firsthand.
    D. restricting communications with other professionals to clinically relevant information.

15. The nurse should use all of the following guidelines for communication with family members EXCEPT:
    A. give information slowly and repeat it as necessary.
    B. answer questions honestly.
    C. use medical terminology.
    D. encourage family members to ask questions.

16. When conflict occurs between the family and the treatment nurse about the child's treatment, the nurse should first:
    A. call the physician and negotiate a change.
    B. contact the home care supervisor.
    C. respect parental preferences if no danger is posed.
    D. explain the correct way and have the family return a demonstration.

17. The nursing process in home care nursing practice integrates:
    A. normalization.
    B. various disciplines.
    C. family priorities.
    D. all of the above.

18. In home nursing practice the nurse strives to help the family maintain control over their:
    A. home.
    B. child's care.
    C. personal lives.
    D. all of the above

19. The school-age child who is physically able may be expected to participate in his/her own care by:
    A. doing no more than holding equipment and discarding used supplies.
    B. administering his/her own medicines with supervision.
    C. assuming responsibility for scheduling home visits.
    D. The school-age child is too young to participate in his/her own care.

20. Laws that ensure that children who are dependent on medical technology are mainstreamed into the school system always result in:
    A. a free, appropriate public education.
    B. payment for health care services in the school setting.
    C. the need for educational planning and coordination.
    D. all of the above.

21. One safety issue that is specific to the home care child who is dependent on electrical equipment is the need to:
    A. have a telephone on-site.
    B. be cared for by trained individuals.
    C. notify telephone and electric companies that the family needs to be placed on a priority service list.
    D. have someone in the house at all times who knows how to perform cardiopulmonary resuscitation.

22. At night the care of the child dependent on medical technology poses the safety concern that:
    A. the child may become frightened from strange noises.
    B. accidental strangulation on equipment wires can occur during sleep.
    C. the lights must be kept brightly lit all night so that procedures can be performed correctly.
    D. all of the above

23. Family-to-family support for the home care child's family:
    A. promotes family strength through shared experiences.
    B. often relieves the health professionals from their role in the primary support system.
    C. meets the specific emotional needs of all families.
    D. all of the above

❖ Critical Thinking ❖
Case Study

William Patterson, who is now 18 months old, was born with Werdnig-Hoffmann disease, a congenital neuromuscular disorder. His disease has developed to the point that he is unable to breathe for more than a few hours without ventilator assistance.

William's older brother George died two years ago from complications of the same disease. His parents took care of him at home until his death. William's parents are preparing for a similar progression of the disease, which means that William will probably be maintained at home on a ventilator for many months until his death.

The case manager assigned to William is the same nurse who was assigned to his brother two years ago. This nurse, Ruth, was instrumental in helping the family cope with the technical issues of home ventilator management and total parenteral nutrition as well as the stressors of caring for their dying child.

24. Ruth is concerned about the boundary between collaborating with the Patterson family and becoming a part of the family as she did when George was dying. She knows that the family is able to technically care for William, but she is feeling as if she also needs to be involved again as part of the family. Ruth has consulted her supervisor for advice. Based on the above information, the supervisor is MOST likely to suggest:
    A. reassignment.
    B. psychological counseling for Ruth.
    C. assessment of therapeutic relationship.
    D. psychological counseling for the Pattersons.

25. At William's stage of development, the home care plan should include ways to promote:
    A. oral-motor development.
    B. mobility and exploration.
    C. self-care.
    D. independence in home management.

26. The quality of William's home care would BEST be evaluated by asking:
    A. Ruth to review the goals.
    B. the Pattersons to review the goals.
    C. Ruth and the Pattersons to jointly review the goals.
    D. the Pattersons to complete an evaluation questionnaire.

❖ Crossword Puzzle ❖

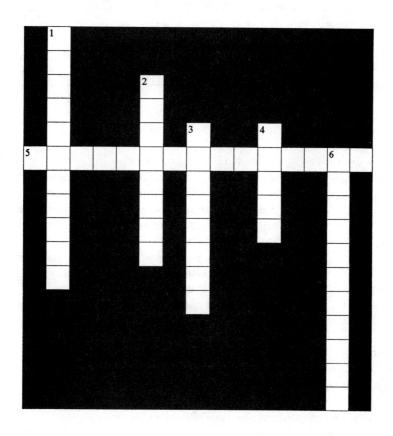

Across

5. Listening beyond the words to hear and understand concerns (2 words)

Down

1. A program of palliative and supportive care services for dying persons and their loved ones (2 words)
2. Care provided for children with complex health care needs in their place of residence (2 words)
3. Exchange of information and sharing of reactions and ideas
4. Listen, Explain, Acknowledge, Recommend, Negotiate
6. The process of examining different options, priorities, and preferences to best meet the needs of the child and family

❖ CHAPTER 26
Family-Centered Care of the Child During Illness and Hospitalization

1. Separation anxiety would be MOST expected in the hospitalized child at age:
   A. 3 to 6 months.
   B. 15 to 30 months.
   C. 30 months to 2 years.
   D. 2 to 4 years.

2. Match the phase of separation anxiety with the behaviors that are typical of that phase.

   A. protest

   B. despair

   C. detachment

   _____ inactive; withdraws from others; uninterested in environment.; uncommunicative; regression behaviors

   _____ interested in surroundings; interacts with caregivers; happy; rarely seen in hospitalized children

   _____ cries; screams; attacks stranger physically and verbally; attempts to escape; continuous crying

3. One difference between the toddler and the school-age child in their reactions to hospitalization is that the school-age child:
   A. does not experience separation anxiety.
   B. has coping mechanisms in place.
   C. relies on his/her family more than the toddler.
   D. experiences separation anxiety to a greater degree.

4. A toddler is most likely to react to short-term hospitalization with feelings of loss of control which are manifested by:
   A. regression.
   B. withdrawal.
   C. formation of new superficial relationships.
   D. self-assertion and anger.

5. The technique of preparing a child for a painful procedure that is specific to the preschool age is to:
   A. encourage the child to act grown up.
   B. demonstrate the procedure.
   C. allow them to participate in the procedure.
   D. allow structured choices.

6. Which one of the following risk factors makes a child more vulnerable to the stressors of hospitalization?
   A. urban dweller
   B. strong-willed
   C. female gender
   D. passive temperament

7. The pediatric population in the hospital today is different from the pediatric population of ten years ago in that the usual length of stay has:
   A. decreased and the acuity has increased.
   B. increased and the acuity has decreased.
   C. increased and the acuity has increased.
   D. decreased and the acuity has decreased.

8. Describe at least one of the possible psychological benefits a child might gain from hospitalization.

   _____

   _____

9. Siblings who visit their brother or sister in the hospital have an increased tendency to exhibit which one of the following behaviors?
   A. nail biting
   B. anger
   C. increased concentration in school
   D. decreased concentration in school

10. Which one of the following statements is TRUE in regard to parent participation in the hospitalized child's care?
    A. The parents need 24-hour responsibility to help maintain their feeling of importance to the child.
    B. Fathers and mothers need the same kind of support during the hospitalization of their child.
    C. Nurses may express support of parent participation but may not foster an environment that encourages parents to stay.
    D. Mothers feel comfortable assuming responsibility for their child's care.

11. To help the parents deal with the issues related to separation while their child is hospitalized, the nurse should NOT suggest:
    A. using associations to help the child understand time frames.
    B. ways to explain departure and return.
    C. quietly leaving while the child is distracted or asleep.
    D. short frequent visits over one extended time if rooming in is impossible.

12. One technique used during hospitalization that can minimize the disruption in the routine of the school-age child who is not critically ill is:
    A. time structuring.
    B. anaclitic care.
    C. self-care.
    D. regulating television viewing.

13. Which one of the following age groups is MOST affected by the hospitalization in regard to their feelings of loss?
    A. infant
    B. toddler
    C. preschooler
    D. school-age child

14. The Joint Commission on Accreditation of Healthcare Organizations recommends that children's rights and responsibilities during the hospitalization be:
    A. the same as those of adults.
    B. the same throughout the agency.
    C. different from those of adults.
    D. prominently displayed as a "Bill of Rights."

15. Preparing children for intrusive procedures usually increases their:
    A. feelings of control.
    B. fear.
    C. stress.
    D. misconceptions.

16. Whenever performing a painful procedure on a child, the nurse should attempt to:
    A. perform the procedure in the playroom.
    B. standardize techniques from one age to the next.
    C. perform the procedure quickly.
    D. have the parents leave during the procedure.

17. After administering an intramuscular injection, the nurse would BEST reassure the young child with poorly defined body boundaries by:
    A. telling the child that the bleeding will stop after the needle is removed.
    B. using a large bandage to cover the injection site.
    C. using a small bandage to cover the injection site.
    D. using a bandage but removing it a few hours after the injection.

18. One way to evaluate whether a child fears mutilation of body parts is to:
    A. explain the procedure.
    B. ask the child to draw a picture of what will happen.
    C. stress the reason for the procedure.
    D. investigate the child's individual concerns.

19. Which of the following reactions to surgery is MOST typical of an adolescent's reaction to fear of bodily injury?
    A. concern about the pain
    B. concern about the procedure itself
    C. concern about the scar
    D. understanding explanations literally

20. In regard to pain assessment, nurses tend to:
    A. underestimate the existence of pain in children but not in adults.
    B. underestimate the existence of pain in both children and adults.
    C. overestimate the existence of pain in children but not in adults.
    D. overestimate the existence of pain in both children and adults.

21. Identify the following statements about pain in children as either TRUE or FALSE.

    _____ Children may not realize how much they are hurting when they are in constant pain.

    _____ Children always tell the truth about pain.

    _____ Narcotics are no more dangerous for children than they are for adults.

    _____ Neonates have the mechanism to transmit noxious stimuli by 20 weeks' gestation.

    _____ Children cannot tell you where they hurt.

    _____ Younger children tend to rate procedure-related pain higher than older children.

    _____ A 3-year-old child can use a pain scale.

    _____ Narcotics are more dangerous for children than for adults.

    _____ Children tolerate pain better than adults.

_____ Children may not admit having pain in order to avoid an injection.

_____ Infants do not feel pain.

_____ Children may believe that the nurse knows how they feel.

_____ Children become accustomed to pain or painful procedures.

_____ Children's signs of discomfort often increase with repeated painful procedures.

_____ The active resistant child will rate pain lower than the passive accepting child.

_____ Addiction from opioids used to treat pain is rare in children.

_____ Respiratory depression in children from opioids is uncommon.

_____ The child's behavior indicates the intensity of the pain.

_____ Infants metabolize opioids in a manner similar to older children.

22. List the six strategies used in the QUESTT approach to pain assessment.

Q _____

U _____

E _____

S _____

T _____

T _____

23. When using Patient Controlled Analgesia (PCA) with children, the:
    A. drug of choice is meperidine.
    B. parent should control the dosing.
    C. nurse should control the dosing.
    D. drug of choice is morphine.

24. The anesthetic cream EMLA is applied:
    A. before invasive procedures.
    B. as preoperative oral sedation.
    C. for chronic cancer pain.
    D. postoperatively.

25. For postoperative or cancer pain control, analgesics should be administered:
    A. as needed.
    B. around the clock.
    C. before the pain escalates.
    D. after the pain peaks.

26. The MOST common side effect from opioid therapy is:
    A. respiratory depression.
    B. pruritus.
    C. nausea and vomiting.
    D. constipation.

27. The treatment of tolerance to opioid therapy includes:
    A. discontinuing the drug.
    B. decreasing the dose.
    C. increasing the dose.
    D. increasing the duration between doses.

28. When choosing play activities for the ill child, it is BEST to select toys that are:
    A. appropriate to the child's developmental age.
    B. simpler than would normally be chosen.
    C. new to cheer and comfort the child.
    D. capable of being disinfected after use.

29. Showing tolerance for deviation from the expected norm when a child is seriously ill:
    A. helps parents accept their feelings.
    B. increases the psychological impact of the illness.
    C. decreases the time it takes for child to adjust.
    D. all of the above

30. Preparation for hospitalization reduces stress in which of the following age groups?
    A. infancy
    B. toddlerhood
    C. preschool
    D. all of the above

31. After hospitalization it is normal for parents to expect the child to:
    A. demand attention.
    B. show signs of regression.
    C. receive a hostile reception from younger siblings.
    D. all of the above

32. Define the role of a child life specialist.

    _____

    _____

    _____

33. Questions related to activities of daily living at the time of admission are:
    A. inappropriate and should be saved for later.
    B. directed toward evaluation of the child's preparation for hospitalization.
    C. asked directly in the order provided on the assessment form.
    D. to help the child adjust to the hospital routines.

34. A benefit of a day hospital is reduction of:
    A. stressors.
    B. infection risk.
    C. cost.
    D. all of the above.

35. The advantages of a hospital unit specifically for adolescents include:
    A. exclusive group membership.
    B. less preparation is needed.
    C. increased socialization with peers.
    D. all of the above.

36. When caring for the child in isolation, the nurse should:
    A. spend as little time as possible in the room.
    B. teach the parents to care for the child to decrease the risk of spreading infection.
    C. let the child see the nurse's face before donning the mask.
    D. all of the above

37. Define *postvention* and describe a situation in which it would be therapeutic.

    _____

    _____

    _____

38. One of the BEST ways to support the parents when they first visit the child in the intensive care unit is:
    A. for the nurse to accompany them to the bedside.
    B. to use picture books of the unit in the waiting area.
    C. to limit the visiting hours so that parents are encouraged to rest.
    D. to expect parents to stay with their child continuously.

39. Transfer from the intensive care unit to the regular pediatric unit can be BEST facilitated by:
    A. discussing the details of the transfer at the bedside where the child can listen.
    B. establishing a schedule that resembles the child's home schedule.
    C. assigning a primary nurse who visits regularly before the transfer.
    D. explaining to the family that there are fewer nurses on the general unit.

40. Transitional care, a trial period for the family to assume the child's care with minimum supervision, may take place:
    A. on the nursing unit.
    B. during a home pass.
    C. in a motel near the hospital.
    D. any of the above

❖ Critical Thinking ❖
Case Study

Peter Chen is an 8-year-old child who is admitted to the pediatric unit for an appendectomy. He is in the third grade and is very active in after-school activities. Recently he began to take karate lessons, and he also plays baseball. He loves school, particularly when he is able to read. Peter awakens every morning at 6 a.m. to read, and reading is the last thing he does before falling asleep.

Peter's parents are with him during the admission interview. His mother works, but she has made arrangements to take some time off during his hospital stay and after the surgery to be available to him.

41. Based on the above information, the nurse should expect:
    A. a normal response to hospitalization.
    B. more anxiety than would normally be seen.
    C. difficulty with the parents.
    D. cultural factors to take precedence.

42. The nurse identifies which of the following nursing diagnoses for Peter?
    A. diversional activity deficit and powerlessness
    B. activity intolerance and high risk for injury
    C. anxiety/fear and self-care deficit
    D. All of the above are possible.

43. One reasonable expected outcome for Peter's diagnosis of powerlessness would be which of the following?
    A. Peter will tolerate increasingly more activity.
    B. Peter will remain injury-free.
    C. Peter will play and rest quietly.
    D. Peter will help plan care and schedule.

44. Which one of the following interventions would be BEST for the nurse to incorporate into Peter's plan?
    A. Organize activities for maximum sleep time.
    B. Keep side rails up.
    C. Choose an appropriate roommate.
    D. Assist with dressing and bathing.

❖ Crossword Puzzle ❖

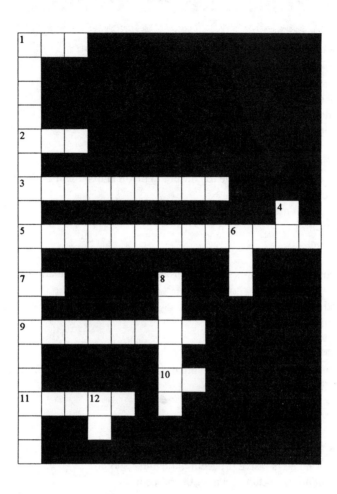

Across

1. Administer as needed
2. Intensive care unit
3. Absence of pain without loss of consciousness
5. Clinical need to increase the drug dosage in order to attain the same desired effect (2 words)
7. Oral
9. Legal term for any substance that causes psychologic dependence
10. Intravenous
11. Nonsteroidal antiinflammatory drug

Down

1. Adaptive physiologic state that occurs when a drug is taken in increasing amounts (2 words)
4. Subcutaneous
6. Around the clock
8. Natural or synthetic analgesic with morphine-like actions
12. Intramuscular

❖ CHAPTER 27
Pediatric Variations of Nursing Interventions

1. An informed consent is required for:
   A. an emergency appendectomy.
   B. a cutdown for intravenous medications.
   C. release of medical information.
   D. all of the above.

2. When the parents are divorced, who is eligible to consent to medical treatment of the child?
   A. Only the custodial parent may consent.
   B. Only the noncustodial parent may consent.
   C. Both parents must consent.
   D. Either parent may consent.

3. The mature minors doctrine permits minors to give consent for treatment in relation to:
   A. psychiatric care.
   B. health care of any kind.
   C. sexually transmitted diseases.
   D. routine physical only.

4. Emancipated minors are usually recognized as having the legal capacity of an adult in all matters after they:
   A. have acquired a sexually transmitted disease.
   B. use contraceptives.
   C. use drugs or alcohol.
   D. become pregnant.

5. If a child needs support during an invasive procedure, the nurse should:
   A. inform the parents about how the child did after the procedure.
   B. ask the parents to stay in the room where they can have eye contact with the child.
   C. decide whether parental presence will be beneficial and try to let the parents choose.
   D. encourage the parents to stay close by to console the child immediately following the procedure.

6. List at least five strategies the nurse can use to support the child during and after a procedure.

   _____

   _____

   _____

   _____

   _____

7. Describe at least one play activity for each of the following procedures.

   A. Ambulation: _____

   B. Range of motion: _____

   C. Injections: _____

   D. Deep breathing: _____

   E. Extending the environment: _____

   F. Soaks: _____

   G. Fluid intake: _____

8. The MOST effective method of preoperative preparation is:
   A. consistent supportive care.
   B. systematic preparation at specific stress points.
   C. offering parents the option of attending the induction of anesthesia.
   D. a single session of preparation.

9. To prepare a breast-fed infant physically for surgery, the nurse would expect to:
   A. permit breast-feeding up to three hours before surgery.
   B. withhold breast-feeding as of midnight the night before surgery.
   C. withhold breast-feeding from four to eight hours before surgery.
   D. replace breast milk with formula and permit feeding up to two hours before surgery.

10. Preoperative sedation in children is BEST accomplished by:
    A. intravenous conscious sedation.
    B. oral transmucosal conscious sedation.
    C. intravenous opioids.
    D. oral analgesics.

11. The BEST choice of premedication for a painful procedure would be:
    A. intramuscular morphine sulfate.
    B. intravenous morphine sulfate through an established site.
    C. intramuscular promethazine, chlorpromazine, and meperidine.
    D. oral promethazine, chlorpromazine, and meperidine.

12. According to the Acute Pain Management Guidelines (1992), meperidine should be used when the patient:
    A. needs chronic dosing.
    B. has impaired renal function.
    C. needs preprocedural sedation.
    D. is allergic to other opioids.

13. Fear of induction of anesthesia by mask can be minimized by applying:
    A. the mask quickly and with assurance.
    B. an opaque mask.
    C. the mask while the child is sitting.
    D. the mask while the child is supine.

14. An increased heart rate, increased respiratory rate, and increased blood pressure in the immediate postoperative period of a young child would MOST likely indicate:
    A. pain.
    B. infection.
    C. increased intracranial pressure.
    D. advanced shock.

15. A change in vital signs of the young child in the postanesthesia recovery room that demands immediate attention is:
    A. increased temperature.
    B. tachycardia.
    C. muscle rigidity.
    D. all of the above.

16. Which one of the following strategies would be considered an organizational attempt to improve compliance of the family with a young child?
    A. incorporating teaching principles that are known to enhance understanding
    B. encouraging the family to adapt to the hospital medication schedules
    C. evaluating and reducing the time the family waits for their appointment
    D. all of the above

17. General guidelines for care of a child's skin would include:
    A. covering the fingers of the extremity used for an intravenous line.
    B. lifting the child under the arms to transfer the child from the bed to a stretcher.
    C. placing a pectin-based skin barrier directly over excoriated skin.
    D. keeping the skin moist at all times.

18. When bathing an uncircumcised male child under the age of 3, the nurse should:
    A. gently remind the child to clean his genital area.
    B. not retract the foreskin.
    C. retract the foreskin.
    D. avoid cleansing between the skinfolds of the genital area.

19. Care for a black child's hair includes braiding the hair:
    A. when it is damp.
    B. tightly.
    C. when it is dry.
    D. after petroleum jelly is applied.

20. To avoid dehydration from diarrhea, the nurse should offer:
    A. gelatin.
    B. plain water.
    C. clear liquids.
    D. fruit juices.

21. Which one of the following examples of a child's food intake would be the BEST sample of adequate documentation?
    A. Child ate one bowl of cereal with milk.
    B. Child ate an adequate breakfast.
    C. Child ate 80% of the breakfast served.
    D. Parent states that child ate an adequate breakfast.

22. The MOST effective intervention for the treatment of fever in a 4-year-old child is to:
    A. administer a tepid sponge bath.
    B. administer ibuprofen.
    C. reduce the room temperature.
    D. administer acetaminophen.

23. The MOST effective intervention for the treatment of hyperthermia in a 4-year-old child is to administer:
    A. a tepid sponge bath.
    B. acetaminophen.
    C. an alcohol sponge bath.
    D. aspirin.

24. Which one of the following recommendations about contamination of the hands during procedures is MOST important for the nurse to adhere to?
    A. Follow disease-specific infection control guidelines.
    B. Wear vinyl gloves.
    C. Avoid wearing nail polish.
    D. Wash the hands routinely after each patient contact.

25. After mouth or lip surgery, the nurse would choose to restrain the child using:
    A. arm and leg restraints.
    B. elbow restraints.
    C. a jacket restraint.
    D. a mummy restraint.

26. The BEST positioning technique for a lumbar puncture in a neonate is a:
    A. side-lying position with neck flexion.
    B. sitting position.
    C. side-lying position with modified neck extension.
    D. side-lying position with knees to chest.

27. The MOST frequently used site for bone marrow aspiration in children is the:
    A. femur.
    B. sternum.
    C. tibia.
    D. iliac crest.

28. To facilitate urination in a 4-year-old child who is toilet trained, the nurse could:
    A. wipe the abdomen with alcohol and fan it dry.
    B. elicit Perez reflex.
    C. apply a urine collection device.
    D. wash and dry the genitalia thoroughly.

29. When applying a urine specimen bag on an infant, it is sometimes necessary to:
    A. oil the surface of the skin.
    B. place the scrotum inside the bag.
    C. remove and replace the bag often.
    D. restrain all four extremities tightly.

30. In order to avoid the complication of necrotizing osteochondritis, the nurse should:
    A. warm the site with moist compresses.
    B. cleanse the site with alcohol.
    C. use an automatic lancet device.
    D. use the inner aspect of the heel.

31. After a venipuncture in the young child, the nurse should:
    A. use "spot" bandage for the day.
    B. extend the arm while pressure is applied.
    C. avoid the use of any bandage.
    D. flex the arm while pressure is applied.

32. To obtain a sputum specimen for tuberculosis or respiratory syncytial virus (RSV) in an infant, the nurse may need to:
    A. have the infant cough.
    B. obtain mucus from the throat.
    C. insert a suction catheter into the back of the throat.
    D. perform gastric lavage.

33. The MOST accurate method for determining the safe dose of a medication for a child is to use:
    A. a Body Surface Area formula.
    B. Clark's rule.
    C. Wright's rule.
    D. milligrams per kilogram.

34. To ensure that medication administration is least traumatic for the child, the nurse should:
    A. administer the drug quickly.
    B. leave the drug with the parent at the bedside.
    C. supervise the parent administering the drug.
    D. ask the parent to assist by restraining the child.

35. To administer 1 teaspoon of medication at home, the BEST device for the nurse to instruct the parent to use would be the:
    A. household soup spoon.
    B. household measuring spoon.
    C. hospital's molded plastic cup.
    D. household teaspoon.

36. All of the following techniques for medication administration to an infant are acceptable EXCEPT:
    A. adding the medication to the infant's formula.
    B. allowing the infant to sit in the parent's lap during administration.
    C. allowing the infant to suck the medication from an empty nipple.
    D. inserting the needleless syringe into the side of the mouth while the infant nurses.

37. When determining the needle length for intramuscular injection of medication into a child, the nurse should:
    A. grasp the muscle and use a length that is half the distance.
    B. use a needle length that is too short rather than one that is too long.
    C. choose a half-inch needle for a 4-month-old infant.
    D. grasp the muscle and use a length that is less than half the distance.

38. Which of the following intramuscular injection sites is generally reserved for children who have been walking for more than a year?
    A. deltoid muscle
    B. vastus lateralis
    C. dorsogluteal
    D. ventrogluteal

39. Describe the difference between the direct technique and the retrograde technique for administering intravenous medications.

_____

_____

_____

40. When administering medications to a child through a gastric tube, the nurse should:
    A. use oily medications to ease passage through the tube.
    B. mix the medication with the enteral formula.
    C. use a syringe with the plunger in place to administer the drug.
    D. flush the tube well between each medication administration.

41. The rectal route of medication administration is used when the child is:
    A. not responding to oral antiemetic preparations.
    B. unable to take anything by mouth.
    C. unlikely to have large amounts of stool.
    D. all of the above

42. To instill eyedrops in an infant whose eyelids are clenched shut, the nurse should:
    A. apply finger pressure to the lacrimal punctum.
    B. place the drops in the nasal corner where the lids meet and wait until the infant opens the lid.
    C. administer the eye drops before nap time.
    D. all of the above

43. During continuous enteral feedings, the nurse should:
    A. use the same pole as the intravenous line.
    B. use a burette to calibrate the feeding times.
    C. give the infant a pacifier for sucking.
    D. all of the above

44. In the small infant, a feeding tube is usually inserted through the:
    A. nose.
    B. mouth.

45. To check the placement of a child's nasogastric tube before each feeding, the nurse should:
    A. aspirate stomach contents and auscultate the stomach for air entry.
    B. place the end of the tube in a glass of water and watch for bubbles with respiration.
    C. aspirate stomach contents and measure the pH.
    D. auscultate the stomach for air entry and obtain an x-ray.

46. One of the major advantages of the recently developed skin level devices for feeding children is that the button device:
    A. does not clog as easily as other devices.
    B. eliminates the need for frequent bubbling.
    C. is less expensive than the traditional devices.
    D. eliminates the need for clamping.

47. When administering an enema to a small child, it is advisable to use:
    A. a pediatric Fleet enema.
    B. a commercially prepared solution.
    C. an isotonic solution.
    D. plain water.

48. A young child with an ostomy pouch may need to:
    A. wear one-piece outfits.
    B. begin toilet training at a later than usual age.
    C. limit activity to avoid skin damage.
    D. use a rubber band to help the appliance fit.

❖ *Critical Thinking* ❖
Case Study

Janis Smith is a 6-year-old child admitted to the hospital for an emergency appendectomy. She is accompanied by her mother. Her parents have been divorced for four years. Janis has a sister who is 7 years old.

49. The nurse's plan for preparing Janis for surgery based on her developmental characteristics should include:
    A. an emphasis on privacy.
    B. the correct scientific medical terminology.
    C. ways to help Janis accept new authority figures.
    D. teaching sessions no longer than five minutes.

50. One of the nursing diagnoses identified by the nurse for Janis is high risk for injury related to the surgical procedure and anesthesia. During the assessment interview, which of the following sets of facts would be MOST pertinent to this diagnosis?
    A. The nurse auscultated vesicular breath sounds.
    B. Janis' mother tells the nurse that the child's father, who is 27 years old and in good health, had some heart problems with anesthesia after a minor surgical procedure last year.
    C. Janis' mother tells the nurse not to expect the child's father to participate in the preoperative preparation because he lives in another state.
    D. The nurse assesses that the child has moist mucous membranes and no tenting of the skin.

51. The nursing diagnosis of anxiety related to the surgery and hospitalization is identified by the nurse. Which one of the following strategies would be BEST for the nurse to incorporate into the surgical care plan to address this diagnosis?
    A. Discuss events that the child remembers.
    B. Administer analgesics around the clock.
    C. Teach the child to use the incentive spirometer.
    D. Ambulate the child as early as possible.

52. To evaluate the care plan in regard to the nursing diagnosis of high risk for fluid volume deficit, the MOST appropriate measurable data that demonstrates that the nurse's goal was met would include the point that:
    A. the child has vesicular breath sounds.
    B. the child's father, who is 27 years old and in good health, had some heart problems with anesthesia after a minor surgical procedure last year.
    C. the child's father lives in another state.
    D. the child has moist mucous membranes and no tenting of the skin.

❖ Crossword Puzzle ❖

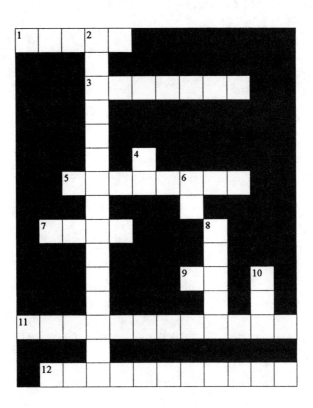

Across

1. Nonsteroidal antiinflammatory drug
3. Pertaining to fever
5. Temperature around which body temperature is regulated (2 words)
7. Postanesthesia care unit
9. Intravenous
11. Body temperature exceeds the set point
12. An agent that relieves or reduces fever

Down

2. Requirement that patient/parents completely understand proposed treatments (2 words)
4. Universal precautions
6. Intramuscular
8. Elevation in set point such that body temperature is regulated at a higher level
10. Body substance isolation

❖ CHAPTER 28
Balance and Imbalance of Body Fluids

1. Match the term with its definition.

   A. total body water   _____ fluid outside the cells

   B. intracellular fluid   _____ fluid within the cells

   C. extracellular fluid   _____ 45% to 75% of body weight

   D. osmotic pressure   _____ enhances sodium reabsorption in renal tubules

   E. diffusion   _____ released from the posterior pituitary gland in response to increased
                                       osmolality and decreased volume of intravascular fluid
   F. aldosterone

                                _____ the physical pull created by a solution of higher concentration
   G. antidiuretic hormone   across a semipermeable membrane

                                _____ random movement of molecules from a region of greater concentra-
                                       tion to regions of lesser concentration

2. The nurse would expect which one of the following conditions to produce an increased requirement?
   A. congestive heart failure
   B. increased intracranial pressure
   C. mechanical ventilation
   D. tachypnea

3. The nurse recognizes which individual as having the LEAST water content in relation to weight?
   A. obese female
   B. thin female
   C. obese male
   D. thin male

4. Infants and young children are at high risk for fluid and electrolyte imbalances. Which one of the following factors
   contributes to this vulnerability?
   A. decreased body surface area
   B. lower metabolic rate
   C. mature kidney function
   D. increased extracellular fluid volume

5. _____ dehydration occurs when electrolyte and water deficits are present in balanced

   proportion.

6. _____ dehydration occurs when the electrolyte deficit exceeds the water deficit. There

   is a greater proportional loss of extracellular fluid, and plasma sodium concentration is usually _____
   than 130 mEq/L.

7. _____ dehydration results from water loss in excess of electrolyte loss. This is often caused by a large _____ of water and/or a large _____ of electrolytes. Plasma sodium concentration is _____ than 150 mEq/L.

8. In infants and young children, the MOST accurate means of describing dehydration or fluid loss is:
   A. as a percentage.
   B. milliliters per kilogram of body weight.
   C. by the amount of edema present or absent.
   D. degree of skin elasticity.

9. An infant with moderate dehydration has what clinical signs?
   A. mottled skin color, decreased pulse and respirations
   B. decreased urine output, tachycardia, fever
   C. tachycardia, oliguria, capillary filling 2-3 seconds
   D. tachycardia, bulging fontanel, decreased blood pressure

10. Johnny, age 13 months, is being admitted for parenteral fluid therapy because of excessive vomiting. The nurse would recognize which one of the following as MOST essential in implementing care for Johnny?
    A. Give Johnny oral fluids until the parenteral fluid therapy can be established.
    B. Question the physician's order for parenteral fluid therapy of glucose 5% in 0.22% sodium chloride.
    C. Withhold the ordered potassium additive until Johnny's renal function has been verified.
    D. Replace half of Johnny's estimated fluid deficit over the first 24 hours of parenteral fluid therapy.

11. Rapid fluid replacement is CONTRAINDICATED in which one of following types of dehydration?
    A. isotonic
    B. hypotonic
    C. hypertonic

12. Water intoxication can occur in children from:
    1. excessive intake of electrolyte-free formula.
    2. administration of inappropriate hypotonic solutions.
    3. dilution of formula with water.
    4. isotonic dehydration.
    5. vigorous hydration with water following a febrile illness.
    6. fluid shifts from intracellular to extracellular spaces.
    A. 1, 2, 3, and 4
    B. 1, 2, 3, and 5
    C. 2, 3, and 4
    D. 2, 3, 5, and 6

13. Severe generalized edema in all body tissues is called _____.

14. Edema formation can be caused by which one of the following?
    A. decreased venous pressure
    B. alteration in capillary permeability
    C. increased plasma proteins
    D. increased tissue tension

15. Match the term with its definition.

A. respiratory acidosis

_____ occurs when there is a reduction of hydrogen ion concentration or an excess of base bicarbonate

B. respiratory alkalosis

_____ caused by any process that reduces base bicarbonate concentration or increases metabolic acid formation

C. metabolic acidosis

D. metabolic alkalosis

_____ results from factors that depress the respiratory center, factors that affect the lung, and factors that interfere with the bellows action of the chest wall

_____ results primarily from central nervous system stimulation

16. To obtain relevant information from the mother of a child with fluid and electrolyte disturbances, the nurse should question the parent about:
A. the type and amount of intake.
B. observations of general appearance.
C. weight of the child.
D. whether the parents have taken the child's temperature within the last 24 hours.

17. Which symptom would the nurse expect in a child with hypocalcemia?
A. abdominal cramps, oliguria
B. muscle cramps, hypertonia
C. thirst, low urine specific gravity
D. flushed, mottled extremities; weight gain

18. Joan, age 3, is admitted for fluid and electrolyte disturbances. The nurse's assessment should include:
1. general appearance observation.
2. vital signs.
3. intake and output measurements.
4. daily weights.
5. review of laboratory results.
A. 1, 2, 3, and 4
B. 2, 3, and 4
C. 3, 4, and 5
D. 1, 2, 3, 4, and 5

19. For encouraging fluid intake and preventing dehydration, the nurse would recommend which one of the following to the parents of 3-year-old Timmy, who has diarrhea?
A. diluted fruit juice
B. decarbonated ginger ale
C. apple juice
D. commercial broth

20. Billy, age 3, has just been ordered NPO. To prevent intake of fluids, the nurse should do which of the following?
A. Place an NPO sign over his bed and remove fluids from the bedside.
B. Place him in a private room away from other children.
C. Apply an elbow restraint jacket to keep Billy from being able to drink by himself.
D. Provide administration of ice chips every 30 minutes.

21. In starting an IV infusion in most children, the nurse recognizes the plan of care should include which of the following?
A. Interruptions during the procedure are kept to a minimum.
B. Use of a 20-gauge over-the-needle catheter is preferred.
C. Allow the child to handle the equipment before procedure.
D. Prepare the IV fluid and tubing after insertion.

22. Identify the following statements about parenteral fluid therapy as either TRUE or FALSE.

_____ Glucose 10% in water is a hypotonic solution.

_____ One molecule of glucose has half the osmolality of one molecule of sodium chloride.

_____ IV solutions given to infants and young children should contain at least 0.2% NaCl to prevent brain edema.

_____ IV infusion for children must be given with an apparatus that delivers a microdrop factor of 60 drops/ml and contains a calibrated volume control chamber.

_____ Pediatric patients receiving IV fluids via continuous infusion pumps need less monitoring.

_____ The IV infusion must be monitored every four hours for proper infusion rate and for site assessment.

23. What nursing action should be included in the plan of care for 10-year-old Debbie, who requires intravenous fluid therapy?
    A. Position the extremity in a natural anatomic position with the fingers and thumb immobilized.
    B. Use opaque covering to secure the IV line, insertion site, and extremity distal to the site.
    C. Teach Debbie how to safely manipulate the IV when getting out of bed and ambulating.
    D. Use Debbie's dominant hand for the IV site if possible.

24. Which one of the following alerts the nurse to a potential problem in a child receiving IV fluids?
    A. edema, blanching, and cool skin at the IV insertion site
    B. The IV tubing is not changed or replaced for 16 hours.
    C. Blood appears in the tubing when the IV bag is held below the IV site level.
    D. unrestricted flushing of the catheter

25. Match the term with its definition. (A term may be used more than once.)

    A. peripheral lock

    B. short-term or nontunneled catheters

    C. short- to moderate-term nontunneled catheters (PICCs)

    D. long-term, tunneled catheters

    _____ includes implanted infusion ports; most contact sports are prohibited

    _____ peripherally inserted central catheters placed by specially trained nurses

    _____ A chest x-ray film should be taken to verify placement of the catheter tip before administration of medication.

    _____ used for intermittent infusion via peripheral route

    _____ If catheter is threaded midline, TPN is not administered because it irritates the vessel.

26. Jamie, age 12, is receiving total parenteral hyperalimentation. The nurse knows that which one of the following serum levels must be carefully monitored?
    A. sodium
    B. calcium
    C. bicarbonate
    D. glucose

❖ Critical Thinking ❖
Case Study

Jennifer, age 4 months, is admitted to the hospital because of dehydration caused by diarrhea. Her mother has been giving her electrolyte-free solutions for volume replacement. Parenteral fluids have been ordered for Jennifer.

27. What type of dehydration does Jennifer MOST likely have?
    A. isotonic
    B. hypertonic
    C. hypotonic
    D. water intoxication

28. Diarrhea MOST commonly causes which one of the following?
    A. respiratory acidosis
    B. respiratory alkalosis
    C. metabolic acidosis
    D. metabolic alkalosis

29. Which of the following questions should the nurse ask in obtaining the admission history?
    A. type of food and fluid intake and amount
    B. urinary output amount or number
    C. number and consistency of stools passed in the past 24 hours
    D. all of the above

30. Which of the following observations does the nurse recognize as the BEST indicator that Jennifer's dehydration is becoming more severe?
    A. Jennifer's cry is whining and low-pitched.
    B. Jennifer's activity level is decreased.
    C. Jennifer's appetite is diminished.
    D. Jennifer is becoming more irritable and lethargic.

❖ *Crossword Puzzle* ❖

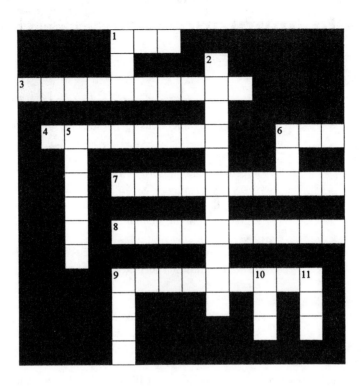

Across

1. Basal metabolic rate
3. Loss of fluid from the body by evaporation and/or respiration
4. Having the same osmotic pressure as a reference solution
6. Total body water
7. Having a greater osmotic pressure than a reference solution
8. Number of particles suspended in fluid
9. Having a lesser osmotic pressure than a reference solution

Down

1. Blood urea nitrogen
2. An element or compound that, when dissolved in a liquid, dissociates into ions and is able to conduct an electric current
5. A substance dissolved in a solution
6. Total parenteral nutrition
9. Home total parenteral nutrition
10. Nothing by mouth
11. Colloidal osmotic pressure

❖ CHAPTER 29
Conditions That Produce Fluid and Electrolyte Imbalance

1. Match the term with its descritption.

A. secretory diarrhea

B. cytotoxic diarrhea

C. osmotic diarrhea

D. dysenteric diarrhea

E. chronic diarrhea

_____ associated with inflammation of the mucosa and submucosa in the ileum and colon by infectious agents such as *Salmonella* or *Shigella*

_____ commonly seen in malabsorption syndrome such as lactose intolerance; the intestine cannot absorb nutrients

_____ usually due to bacterial enterotoxins which stimulate fluid and electrolyte secretion from the small intestine

_____ viral destruction of the mucosal cells within the small intestine resulting in a smaller intestinal surface area and decreased absorption of fluid and electrolytes

_____ may be the result of inadequate management of acute diarrhea; increase in stool frequency and increased water content with a duration of more than 14 days

2. The nurse recognizes that which one of the following is MOST likely to develop acute diarrhea?
   A. the 2-month-old infant who attends day care each day
   B. the 18-month-old infant who stays at home each day with his mother
   C. the 6-year-old child who attends public school
   D. the 24-month-old infant with two older brothers, ages 5 years and 8 years

3. Identify the following statements as either TRUE or FALSE.

_____ Rotavirus is the most common pathogen identified in young children in this country hospitalized for diarrhea and dehydration.

_____ Acute diarrhea in children may be associated with respiratory infections, otitis media infections, and urinary tract infections.

_____ Excessive ingestion of apple juice can cause osmotic dietary diarrhea.

_____ Ampicillin, amoxicillin, cephalothin, and cefaclor are seldom associated with diarrhea in children because of their lower specific gravity.

_____ *Clostridium difficile* produces a protective mechanism against diarrhea because it alters the intestinal flora, increasing absorption surfaces.

_____ Because the infant's metabolic rate is lower than the adult's metabolic rate, the infant is more rapidly depleted of nutritional reserves during periods of malabsorption and decreased intake and therefore more prone to the development of dehydration.

4. Johnny, age 2 years, is diagnosed with uncomplicated diarrhea with no signs of dehydration. Diagnostic evaluation should include which one of the following?
   A. cultures of the stool
   B. presence of associated symptoms
   C. complete blood count
   D. urine specific gravity

5. A priority goal in the management of acute diarrhea is:
   A. determining the cause of the diarrhea.
   B. preventing the spread of the infection.
   C. rehydration of the child.
   D. managing the fever associated with the diarrhea.

6. The MOST appropriate therapeutic management for rehydration of Jenny, age 8 months, who has been diagnosed with acute diarrhea and has evidence of mild dehydration, is:
   A. oral rehydration therapy of 50 ml/kg within four hours.
   B. restarting lactose-free formula.
   C. encouraging intake of clear fluids by mouth, such as fruit juices and gelatin.
   D. BRAT diet, which consists of bananas, rice, apples, and toast or tea.

7. Drug therapy for acute infectious diarrhea in young children should include:
   A. Kaopectate administered until the diarrhea has stopped.
   B. continuation of antibiotics for the presence of *C. difficile*.
   C. administration of sedatives to decrease bowel motility.
   D. antibiotic therapy based on culture results.

8. Which one of the following nursing interventions is NOT appropriate for 6-month-old Terry, admitted to the pediatric unit with acute diarrhea and vomiting?
   A. ongoing assessment of Terry's intake and output and physical appearance
   B. education of the parents about the necessity of oral rehydration solution administration
   C. rectal temperatures at least every four hours to monitor fever elevations
   D. gentle cleansing of perianal areas and application of protective topical ointments

9. Therapeutic management of chronic nonspecific diarrhea includes:
   A. high-fructose diet.
   B. increased fiber in the diet.
   C. low-fat diet.
   D. increase of total fluid intake.

10. The major emphasis of nursing care for the vomiting infant or child is:
    A. observation and reporting of vomiting behavior.
    B. observation and reporting of associated symptoms of vomiting.
    C. implementation of measures to reduce the vomiting.
    D. all of the above.

11. Fill in the blanks in the following statements.

    A. _____ shock follows a reduction in circulating blood volume, plasma volume, or extra-cellular fluid loss.

    B. _____ shock results from impaired cardiac muscle function, resulting in reduced cardiac output.

    C. _____ shock results from a vascular abnormality that produces maldistribution of blood supply throughout the body.

D. _____ shock is characterized by a hypersensitivity reaction causing massive vasodilation and capillary leak.

E. _____ shock is characterized by a decreased cardiac output and derangements in the peripheral circulation in response to a severe, overwhelming infection.

12. Clinical manifestations of pronounced tachycardia, narrowed pulse pressure, poor capillary filling, and increased confusion would suggest which of the following?
    A. compensated shock
    B. decompensated shock
    C. irreversible shock

13. Match the stage of septic shock with its characteristics.

    A. hyperdynamic stage   _____   lasts for only a few hours with respiratory distress, narrow pulse pressure, severe hypotension, profound hypothermia

    B. normodynamic stage

                                   _____   warm, flushed skin with tachypnea, chills, and fever, and normal urinary
    C. hypodynamic stage   output

                                   _____   cool shock with depressed sensorium, oliguria, slightly elevated systemic blood pressure, cool extremities, and normal pulses

14. The MOST common initial sign of anaphylaxis is:
    A. cutaneous manifestations; the child may complain of feeling warm.
    B. bronchiolar constriction with wheezing.
    C. vasodilation and hypotension.
    D. laryngeal edema and stridor.

15. In teaching adolescent females how to prevent toxic shock syndrome, the nurse includes which one of the following as the BEST mechanism of prevention?
    A. Remove the tampon with symptoms of sudden fever, vomiting, diarrhea, or muscle pain.
    B. Wash hands before insertion of the tampon.
    C. Use tampons only during the day; use napkin at night.
    D. Avoid the use of tampons.

16. Burns are caused by _____, _____, _____,

    and _____ agents.

17. _____ burns are the most common cause of burn injuries in children under the age

    of 3. The 3- to 8-year-old group is more frequently involved with burns from _____

    _____.

18. Identify the following statements as either TRUE or FALSE.

    _____   The single most important factor in the decrease in fire-related deaths since 1978 is the use of smoke detectors.

    _____   Since electric current travels through the body on the path of least resistance, the area surrounding long bones would be expected to experience the most damage.

    _____   An area of concern for electrical burns in the very young child is chewing on electrical cords.

_____ The physiologic responses, therapy, prognosis, and disposition of the injured child with burns are all directly related to the amount of tissue destroyed.

19. The standard adult rule of nines cannot be utilized to determine the total body surface area of a burn in a child because:
    A. the child has different body proportions than the adult.
    B. the child has different fluid body weight than the adult.
    C. the child's proportions of trunk and arms are larger than the adult's.
    D. as the infant grows, percentage for head increases while percentage for arms decreases.

20. Burns involving the epidermis and part of the dermis that exhibit blister and edema formation and that are extremely sensitive to temperature changes, exposure to air, and light touch are termed:
    A. superficial first-degree burns.
    B. partial-thickness second-degree burns.
    C. full-thickness third-degree burns.
    D. fourth-degree burns.

21. The severity of the burn injury is NOT determined by which one of the following?
    A. the intensity of the heat source and the duration of the contact with the causative agent
    B. the causative agent of the burn
    C. the age of the victim
    D. early debridement of burn tissue

22. The nurse recognizes that which one of the following pediatric clients is at higher risk of complications from burn injury?
    A. the 12-month-old infant who pulled hot water over on his chest
    B. the 12-month-old infant who is burned on his chest by gasoline
    C. the 9-month-old infant who is burned on the hands and feet with scalding water as a punishment
    D. the 12-year-old child who is burned on one side of the face as a result of playing with cigarettes

23. Which instruction should be included in the teaching plan for emergency care of the burned child?
    A. Stop the burning process for burns with large amounts of denuded skin by application of large amounts of cool water.
    B. Apply ointments to the burned area before transfer of the child.
    C. Remove jewelry and metal.
    D. Apply neutralizing agents to the skin of chemical burn areas.

24. Which instruction should NOT be included in the teaching plan for the parents of Johnny, age 2 years, who has suffered a minor burn injury?
    A. Wash the wound twice daily with mild soap and tepid water.
    B. Soak the dressing in tepid water before removal to reduce discomfort.
    C. Administer acetaminophen immediately after each dressing change.
    D. Watch the wound margins for redness, edema, or purulent drainage.

25. In major burn injuries of children weighing less than 30 kg, adequate fluid replacement during the emergent phase is BEST assessed by which one of the following?
    A. maintaining an hourly urinary output of 30 ml per hour
    B. urinary output of 1 to 2 ml/kg per hour
    C. increasing hematocrit
    D. normal capillary refill

26. The child with a major burn injury requires which one of the following nutrition plans?
    A. high-protein, high-caloric diet
    B. vitamin A and C supplements
    C. supplements of zinc
    D. all of the above

27. Johnny, age 8 years, suffered partial-thickness second-degree burns of his chest, abdomen, and upper legs while on a recent camping trip. He is scheduled for hydrotherapy each morning for 20 minutes followed by debridement of the wounds. The BEST nursing action to assist Johnny at this time would be which of the following?
   A. Ensure that pain medication is given before hydrotherapy.
   B. Hold Johnny's breakfast until he returns from treatment.
   C. Offer sedation after the procedure to promote rest.
   D. Reassure Johnny that hydrotherapy is not painful.

❖ Critical Thinking ❖
Case Study

Kenny, age 5 years, is brought to the emergency center after his clothes caught on fire while he was playing in the family garage with matches. He has partial-thickness second-degree burns and full-thickness third-degree burns of his anterior chest, anterior abdomen, upper right arm, both shoulders, and right hand. There is singed nasal hair apparent on physical examination and some minor burns apparent on his face. A Foley catheter is inserted and a small amount of clear urine is obtained. Two IV routes are established for fluid replacement.

28. In conducting the physical examination of Kenny's burns, the nurse calculates the extent of body surface area involvement. How would the nurse BEST assess to see if circulation to the area is intact?
   A. Touch the area to see if Kenny feels pain.
   B. Test injured surfaces for blanching and capillary refill.
   C. Inspect the burns for eschar formation.
   D. Watch for edema of the affected part.

29. Based on the information given, the nurse would be careful to watch Kenny for immediate signs of which complication?
   A. inhalation injury
   B. facial deformities
   C. sepsis
   D. renal failure related to formation of myoglobin

30. Kenny has normal bowel sounds 24 hours following admission and is placed on a high-caloric, high-protein diet of which he eats very little. Kenny's hydrotherapy is scheduled right after breakfast and before supper. Which one of the following interventions by the nurse would MOST likely increase Kenny's dietary intake?
   A. Show Kenny a feeding tube and explain to him that if he does not eat more the tube will need to be inserted.
   B. Maintain the current meal schedule and stay with Kenny until he eats all of his meal.
   C. Rearrange his meal and hydrotherapy schedule to prevent conflicts.
   D. Insist that Kenny stop snacking between meals.

31. Considering the extent and distribution of Kenny's burns, which one of the following nursing diagnoses would be recognized as having the highest priority for Kenny during the management phase of his illness?
   A. impaired gas exchange related to inhalation injury
   B. high risk for altered nutrition: less than body requirements related to loss of appetite
   C. fluid volume deficit related to edema associated with burn injury
   D. high risk for infection related to denuded skin, presence of pathogenic organisms, and altered immune response

32. Kenny progressed well with skin grafts and healing and is now ready for discharge. The nurse will know that Kenny's parents understand discharge instructions by which one of the following statements?
   A. "Kenny will need to wear this elastic support bandage for only one month."
   B. "Kenny will not be able to participate in any sports until the grafts have taken hold firmly."
   C. "We will visit the teacher and Kenny's peers before Kenny returns to school to prepare them for his appearance."
   D. "We will need to protect Kenny from normal activities until he requires no further surgery."

❖ Crossword Puzzle ❖

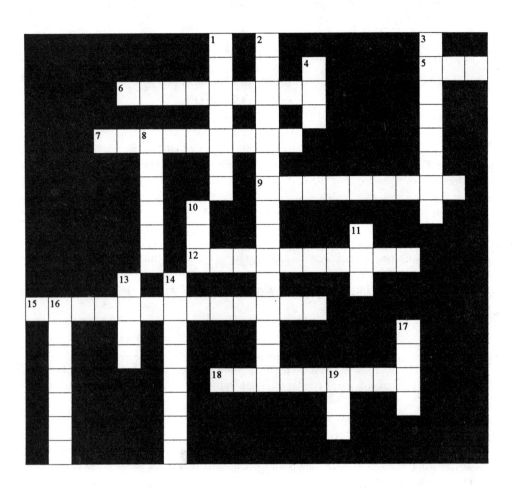

Across

5. Central nervous system
6. Serum pH equal to or greater than 7.45
7. Intestinal inflammation accompanied by cramping, abdominal pain, tenesmus, and watery stools
9. Inflammation of the intestine
12. By some means other than through the digestive tract
15. Return of undigested food from the stomach
18. Inflammation of the stomach

Down

1. Inflammation of the colon
2. Inflammation of the stomach and intestines
3. Serum pH equal to or less than 7.35
4. Toxic shock syndrome
8. Relating to or caused by sepsis
10. Central venous pressure
11. Oral rehydration solution
13. Adult respiratory distress syndrome
14. Increase in number and/or consistency of stools
16. By way of the alimentary tract
17. Chronic nonspecific diarrhea
19. Intracranial pressure

❖ CHAPTER 30
The Child with Renal Dysfunction

1. Identify the following statements as either TRUE or FALSE.

_____ The primary responsibility of the kidney is to maintain the composition and volume of body fluids in excess of body needs.

_____ The kidney functions in the production of erythropoietin and thus in the formation of red blood cell production.

_____ Renin is secreted by the kidney in response to reduced blood volume, decreased blood pressure, or increased secretion of catecholamines.

_____ Approximately one-half of the total cardiac output makes up the blood flow to the kidneys.

_____ Protein is a normal finding in urine because it is too large a molecule to be reabsorbed in the proximal tubule.

_____ Glucose is reabsorbed in the proximal tubule and returned directly to the blood.

_____ Because there is a limit to the concentration gradient against which sodium can be transported out, when larger than normal amounts of sodium remain in the tubules, water is obliged to remain with the sodium.

_____ An end product of protein metabolism is urea.

_____ The newborn is unable to dispose of excess water and solute efficiently because glomerular filtration and absorption do not reach adult values until the child is between 1 and 2 years of age.

_____ The loop of Henle, the site of urine-concentrating mechanism, is short in the newborn, thus reducing the ability to reabsorb sodium and water and produce a concentrated urine output.

_____ Newborn infants are unable to excrete a water load at rates similar to those of older persons.

_____ The abnormal or backward urine movement is termed *reflux*.

2. Jordan is a 2-year-old who had a clean-catch urinalysis done as part of a diagnostic work-up. Match the following results with the nurse's correct interpretation. (Answers may be used more than once.)

A. normal   _____   +1 Glucose

B. abnormal   _____   Specific gravity 1.020

                         _____   RBC 3-4

                         _____   WBC 10

                         _____   Occasional casts

                         _____   Trace protein

                         _____   + Nitrites

3. The nurse, in preparing the child for a diagnostic test, explains that which one of the following tests provides direct visualization of the bladder through a small scope?
A. cystoscopy
B. voiding cystourethrogram
C. IVP
D. renal biopsy

4. Preprocedural preparation of the child who is scheduled to have a cystourethrography includes:
A. keeping the child NPO for eight hours before the test.
B. assessing for an allergy to iodine.
C. administering a Fleet enema before the examination.
D. preparing the child for catheterization.

5. Which one of the following does NOT predispose the client to urinary tract infections?
A. the short urethra in the young female
B. the presence of urinary stasis
C. urinary reflux
D. lowering of urine pH

6. Which symptom suggests pyelonephritis in a 3-year-old child?
A. flank pain and tenderness
B. foul-smelling urine
C. dysuria or urgency
D. enuresis or daytime incontinence

7. The nurse is requested to obtain a urine specimen from 5-year-old Anne. Which of the following methods is the CORRECT procedure?
A. Place a urine bag on Anne to collect the next specimen.
B. Obtain a clean-catch specimen.
C. Encourage Anne to drink large volumes of water in an attempt to obtain a specimen.
D. Obtain a midstream specimen, preferably the first morning specimen.

8. Justin, age 8 years, has been diagnosed with pyelonephritis. The nurse would expect medical management to include:
A. administration of oral nitrofurantoin.
B. admission to the hospital with intravenous antibiotics administered for the first 24 hours.
C. radiographic evaluation.
D. urine cultures repeated every month for three months.

9. The nurse is developing a preventive teaching plan for Tracy, a sexually active 16-year-old who was diagnosed with a urinary tract infection. Which one of the following does the nurse include in the plan?
   A. Promote perineal hygiene by wiping back to front.
   B. Avoid constipation.
   C. Douche as soon as possible after intercourse to flush out bacteria.
   D. Eliminate all carbonated and caffeinic beverages because they irritate the bladder.

10. Vesicoureteral reflux is closely associated with which one of the following?
    A. acute glomerulonephritis
    B. nephrotic syndrome
    C. renal scarring and kidney damage
    D. urinary tract infections caused by high alkaline content

11. Which one of the following clinical manifestations is associated with acute glomerulonephritis?
    A. normal blood pressure, generalized edema, oliguria
    B. periorbital edema, hypertension, hematuria, azotemia
    C. fatigue, elevated serum lipid levels, elevated serum protein levels
    D. temperature elevation, circulatory congestion, normal BUN and creatinine serum levels

12. Which one of the following is an important nursing intervention in caring for the child with acute glomerulonephritis?
    A. enforced bed rest
    B. daily weights
    C. water restriction
    D. low-protein diet

13. Clinical manifestations of nephrotic syndrome include:
    A. hypercholesterolemia, hypoalbuminemia, edema, and proteinuria.
    B. hematuria, hypertension, periorbital edema, and flank pain.
    C. oliguria, hypocholesterolemia, and hyperalbuminemia.
    D. hematuria, generalized edema, hypertension, and proteinuria.

14. Therapeutic management in nephrotic syndrome includes the administration of prednisone. The nurse teaches which of the following as CORRECT administration guidelines?
    A. Corticosteroid therapy is begun after BUN and serum creatinine elevation.
    B. Prednisone is administered orally in a dosage of 4 mg/kg of body weight.
    C. After the child is free of proteinuria and edema, the daily dose of prednisone is gradually tapered over several weeks to months.
    D. The drug is discontinued as soon as the urine is free from protein.

15. Identify the following statements as either TRUE or FALSE.

    _____ Proximal tubular acidosis is caused by the inability of the kidney to establish a normal pH gradient between tubular cells and tubular contents.

    _____ Primary functions of the distal renal tubules are acidification of urine, potassium secretion, and selective and differential reabsorption of sodium, chloride, and water.

    _____ Treatment of both proximal and distal disorders consists of administration of sufficient bicarbonate or citrate to balance metabolically produced hydrogen ions and maintain the plasma bicarbonate level within normal range.

    _____ In nephrogenic diabetes insipidus, the distal tubules and collecting ducts are insensitive to the action of antidiuretic hormone and vasopressin.

    _____ Nephrogenic diabetes insipidus occurs primarily in females and appears in the newborn period with vomiting, fever, failure to thrive, dehydration, and hypernatremia.

_____ Hemolytic-uremic syndrome is characterized by acute renal failure, hemolytic anemia, and thrombocytopenia.

_____ Alport syndrome is a syndrome of chronic hereditary nephritis which consists of hematuria, high-frequency sensorineural deafness, ocular disorders, and chronic renal failure.

_____ Transient proteinuria generally means renal disease.

16. In the evaluation of the child with possible renal trauma, which one of the following is usually indicative of kidney damage?
    A. flank pain and hematuria
    B. dysuria, proteinuria, and nausea
    C. abdominal ascites, nausea, and hematuria
    D. proteinuria and bladder spasms

17. The MOST frequent cause of prerenal failure in infants and children is:
    A. nephrotoxic agents.
    B. obstructive uropathy.
    C. dehydration related to diarrhea and vomiting.
    D. burn shock.

18. The primary manifestation of acute renal failure is:
    A. edema.
    B. oliguria.
    C. metabolic acidosis.
    D. weight gain and proteinuria.

19. The MOST immediate threat to the life of the child with acute renal failure is:
    A. hyperkalemia.
    B. anemia.
    C. hypertensive crisis.
    D. cardiac failure from hypovolemia.

20. Drug therapy utilized for the removal of potassium is:
    A. furosemide.
    B. glucose, 50% and insulin.
    C. Kayexalate.
    D. calcium gluconate.

21. Which one of the following manifestations of chronic renal failure may have the MOST social consequences for the developing child?
    A. anemia
    B. growth retardation
    C. bone demineralization
    D. septicemia

22. Dietary regulation in the child with chronic renal failure includes:
    A. restriction of protein intake below the recommended daily allowance.
    B. to include protein in the diet of high biologic value.
    C. restriction of potassium when creatinine clearance falls below 50 ml/min.
    D. vitamin A, E, and K supplements.

23. Fill in the blanks in the following statements.

A. Methods of dialysis for management of renal failure are _____, _____

_____, and _____.

B. _____ is the preferred method for children with life-threatening hyperkalemia.

C. In peritoneal dialysis, _____ _____ is greater than with hemodialysis.

D. _____ is not recommended for small children because of the rapid changes in blood volume and systemic blood pressure and the difficulty of placing vascular access devices.

E. The major complication associated with peritoneal dialysis is _____.

F. The nurse can expect to see the child undergoing dialysis to have improved _____

_____ and _____ _____ but not to recover to

_____ _____.

G. Continuous arteriovenous hemofiltration is an ideal form of dialysis for children with _____

_____ from _____ _____.

24. Johnny, age 12, had a renal transplant five months ago. He now presents to the hospital outpatient clinic with fever, tenderness over the graft area, decreased urinary output, and a slightly elevated blood pressure. The nurse's priority at this time is:
A. to recognize that Johnny is probably undergoing acute rejection and to notify the physician immediately.
B. to recognize that this is an episode of increased inflammation within the donor kidney because Johnny has probably been noncompliant with his immunosuppressant drugs.
C. to obtain a urine for culture and sensitivity and a blood count to quickly identify Johnny's infection before alerting the physician.
D. to recognize that Johnny is in chronic rejection and that no present therapy can halt the progressive process.

❖ Critical Thinking ❖
Case Study

Dean, age 3 years, is brought to the clinic by his mother. He has a history of a recent fever of 100.2° F, sore throat, and slight cough approximately eight days ago that lasted about three days. Yesterday morning his mother noticed "puffiness around his eyes" when he got up and then "swelling of his lower legs and scrotal area." Dean's appetite and activity level have decreased. This morning Dean's mother noticed that his urine was "darker in color" and "seemed to be smaller in volume." Physical examination reflects a child who does not appear acutely ill but who is irritable and appears fatigued, with pallor. His blood pressure, pulse, and temperature are within normal limits. He has generalized edema. Laboratory findings of his urine specimen include large amounts of protein and microscopic hematuria. Serum protein levels are very low, with elevated lipid levels.

25. Based on the above information, the nurse would suspect that Dean has developed which one of the following conditions?
A. acute poststreptococcal glomerulonephritis
B. minimal-change nephrotic syndrome
C. acute renal failure
D. hemolytic-uremic syndrome

26. Dean is diagnosed by the health care provider as having nephrotic syndrome. Identify goals for restoring renal function in Dean.
    1. Urine is protein-free.
    2. Edema is resolved.
    3. Fluid and electrolyte balance are restored.
    4. Nutritional needs have returned to a state of positive nitrogen balance.
    A. 1, 2, and 3
    B. 1, 2, and 4
    C. 2 and 3
    D. 1, 2, 3, and 4

27. Which one of the following nursing diagnoses is of LEAST benefit in planning for Dean's care?
    A. impaired skin integrity related to edema, lowered body defenses
    B. altered nutrition: less than body requirements related to decreased appetite
    C. altered patterns of elimination related to obstruction
    D. fluid volume excess related to fluid accumulation in tissues and third space

28. Which nursing intervention is appropriate for Dean's nursing diagnosis of impaired skin integrity?
    A. Administer corticosteroids on time with careful monitoring for infections.
    B. Monitor for complications, strict intake and output, daily checks of urine for protein, daily weight, and abdominal girth.
    C. Enforce bed rest during the edema phase of the disease.
    D. Support scrotum on small pillow.

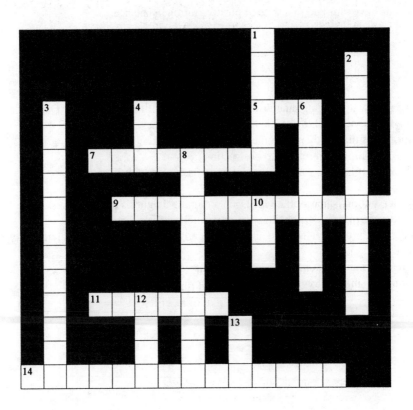

Across

5. Renal tubular acidosis
7. Diminished output of urine
9. Abnormal potassium concentration in the blood
11. Presence of excessive amounts of urea and other nitrogenous wastes in the blood
14. Defective bone formation

Down

1. Absence of urine formation
2. Growth of bacteria in uncontaminated urine
3. Dialysis in which blood is circulated outside the body through artificial membranes
4. Urinary tract infection
6. Excessive amounts of nitrogenous compounds in the blood
8. Inflammation of the urethra
10. Acute renal failure
12. End-stage renal disease
13. Vesicoureteral reflux

❖ CHAPTER 31
The Child with Disturbance of Oxygen and Carbon Dioxide Exchange

1. The general shape of the chest at birth is:
   A. relatively round.
   B. flattened from side to side.
   C. flattened from front to back.
   D. the same shape as an adult's.

2. The infant relies primarily on:
   A. mouth breathing.
   B. intercostal muscles for breathing.
   C. diaphragmatic abdominal breathing.
   D. all of the above.

3. Because of the position of the diaphragm in the newborn:
   A. there is additional abdominal distention from gas and fluid in the stomach.
   B. the diaphragm does not contract as forcefully as that of an older infant or child.
   C. diaphragmatic fatigue is uncommon.
   D. lung volume is increased.

4. Which one of the following statements is TRUE in regard to the anatomy of an infant's nasopharyngeal area?
   A. The glottis is located deeper in infants than in older children.
   B. The laryngeal reflexes are weaker in infants than in older children.
   C. The epiglottis is longer and projects more posteriorly in infants than in adults.
   D. The infant and young child are both less susceptible than adults to edema formation in the nasopharyngeal regions.

5. List four anatomical factors that significantly affect the development of respiratory disorders in infants.

   _____

   _____

   _____

   _____

6. Which one of the following conditions will reduce the number of alveoli?
   A. maternal heroine use
   B. increased prolactin
   C. hyperthyroidism
   D. kyphoscoliosis

7. As the child grows, chest wall compliance (circle one) INCREASES or DECREASES.

8. As the child grows, elastic recoil of the lungs (circle one) INCREASES or DECREASES.

9. Relaxation of the bronchial smooth muscles occurs in response to:
   A. parasympathetic stimulation.
   B. inhalation of irritating substances.
   C. sympathetic stimulation.
   D. histamine release.

10. Room air consists of:
    A. 7% oxygen.
    B. 21% oxygen.
    C. 50% oxygen.
    D. 79% oxygen.

11. A child with anemia tends to be fatigued and breathes more rapidly because the majority of oxygen is carried through the blood as:
    A. a solute dissolved in the plasma and water of the red blood cell.
    B. bicarbonate and hydrogen ions.
    C. carbonic acid.
    D. oxyhemoglobin.

12. Retractions are defined as:
    A. the sinking in of soft tissues during the respiratory cycle.
    B. proliferation of the tissue near the terminal phalanges.
    C. increases in the end-expiratory pressure.
    D. results from contraction of the sternocleidomastoid muscles.

13. In a child, cough may be absent in the early stages of:
    A. cystic fibrosis.
    B. measles.
    C. pneumonia.
    D. croup.

14. Match the diagnostic test with the information the test measures.

    A. arterial blood gas   _____ photometric measurement of O_2 saturation (SaO_2)

    B. oximetry   _____ a sequence of pictures, each representing a cross section of or cut
                                                          through lung tissue at a different depth

    C. transcutaneous CO_2 monitoring
                                                    _____ a sensitive indicator to monitor O_2, CO_2, and pH

    D. radiography
                                                    _____ clearly identifies soft tissues with a two- or three-dimensional image

    E. magnetic resonance imaging
                                                    _____ produces images of internal structures of the chest, including air-
    F. computerized tomography   filled lungs, vascular markings, heart, and great vessels

                                                    _____ provides a noninvasive continuous and reliable measurement of
                                                          arterial carbon dioxide

15. When caring for the infant who is connected to a pulse oximeter, the nurse should:
    A. heat the skin.
    B. attach the transducer very tightly.
    C. tape the sensor securely to the great toe.
    D. use a finger cot to cover the sensor.

16. The nurse performs a precautionary assessment of the collateral circulation whenever anyone performs an arterial puncture on the child. This test is called the:
    A. cover test.
    B. Allen test.
    C. Miller test.
    D. Weber test.

17. Oxygen delivered to infants is BEST tolerated when it is administered:
    A. directly in the face of the infant under a hood.
    B. by a hood that extends to touch the infant's shoulders.
    C. by an oxygen tent that does not come into direct contact with the face.
    D. by a hood that can maintain either a low or a high concentration of O_2.

18. The oxygen mist tent is used for MOST children past early infancy who need oxygen, because the oxygen mist tent:
    A. comes into direct contact with the face.
    B. controls and maintains the oxygen above 50%.
    C. is the most comfortable device for children.
    D. keeps the child warm and dry.

19. When caring for the child receiving oxygen via a mist tent, the nurse should:
    A. encourage the child to have a stuffed animal in the tent.
    B. open the tent as little as possible.
    C. open the tent at the bottom of the bed to allow as little oxygen to escape as possible.
    D. keep the child cool because the tent becomes very warm.

20. Oxygen-induced CO_2 narcosis is encountered MOST frequently in children with:
    A. prematurity.
    B. asthma.
    C. cystic fibrosis.
    D. congenital heart disease.

21. For a child under the age of 5 who needs intermittent delivery of an aerosolized medication, the nurse should consider using a:
    A. hand-held nebulizer.
    B. metered-dose inhaler with a spacer device.
    C. humidified mist tent with low-flow oxygen.
    D. metered-dose inhaler without a spacer device.

22. Postural drainage should be performed:
    A. before meals but following other respiratory therapy.
    B. after meals but before other respiratory therapy.
    C. before meals and before other respiratory therapy.
    D. after meals and after other respiratory therapy.

23. Which of the following children would need special modifications of the usual postural drainage techniques?
    A. infants
    B. children with head injuries
    C. children in traction
    D. all of the above

24. Which of the following techniques of chest physiotherapy have been shown through research to be effective modalities?
    A. postural drainage with forced expiration
    B. postural drainage with percussion
    C. percussion and vibration
    D. all of the above

25. The BEST method to stimulate deep breathing in children is to:
    A. encourage the child to cover the mouth and suppress the cough.
    B. encourage the child to cough repeatedly.
    C. use games that extend expiratory time and pressure.
    D. leave some balloons at the bedside for the child to blow up.

26. When using the bag-valve-mask device, the nurse should:
    A. use the device without a reservoir.
    B. use the device with a reservoir.
    C. use a low oxygen concentration.
    D. hyperextend the child's neck.

27. The MOST severe complication that can occur during the intubation procedure is:
    A. infection.
    B. sore throat.
    C. laryngeal stenosis.
    D. hypoxia.

28. When suctioning the airway in a child, the vacuum pressure should range from:
    A. 30 to 50 mm Hg.
    B. 50 to 80 mm Hg.
    C. 80 to 100 mm Hg.
    D. 110 to 120 mm Hg.

29. When suctioning a child's airway, the nurse should NOT:
    A. use continuous suction.
    B. inject any saline into the tube.
    C. insert the catheter into the end of the tube.
    D. use intermittent suction.

30. Suctioning in a child should require no more than:
    A. 3 seconds.
    B. 5 seconds.
    C. 8 seconds.
    D. 10 seconds.

31. Which of the following tracheostomy dressings would be unacceptable?
    A. hydrocolloid wafers
    B. Allevyn dressing
    C. a 4 x 4 gauze pad cut into the needed shape
    D. Hollister Restore

32. After the initial postoperative change, the tracheostomy tube is usually changed:
    A. weekly by the surgeon.
    B. weekly by the nurse.
    C. monthly by the surgeon.
    D. monthly by the family.

33. A tracheostomy with a speaking valve:
    A. decreases secretions.
    B. decreases the child's sense of taste and smell.
    C. limits gas exchange.
    D. has no effect on the ability to swallow.

34. List at least ten conditions that would predispose a child to respiratory failure.

_____   _____

_____   _____

_____   _____

_____   _____

_____   _____

35. Which one of the following contains the early subtle signs of hypoxia?
    A. peripheral cyanosis
    B. central cyanosis
    C. hypotension
    D. mood changes and restlessness

36. Close continuous monitoring of the child with respiratory distress should be used to control the oxygen demands of the body by all of the following methods EXCEPT:
    A. maintaining temperature within normal limits.
    B. placing the child in supine position.
    C. controlling pain.
    D. maintaining an ambient room temperature.

37. Cardiac arrest in the pediatric population is MOST often a result of:
    A. atherosclerosis.
    B. congenital heart disease.
    C. prolonged hypoxia.
    D. undiagnosed cardiac conditions.

38. The first action for the nurse to take when a child has an emergency outside the hospital is to:
    A. transport the child to an acute care facility.
    B. determine whether the child is unconscious.
    C. administer rescue breathing.
    D. transport the child by car for help.

39. At what age range would the nurse place the bag-valve-mask over both the mouth and the nose?
    A. birth to 1 year
    B. 1 year to 3 years
    C. birth to 3 years
    D. birth to 2 years

40. At what age range in an emergency situation should the nurse assess circulation by palpating the carotid pulse?
    A. 1 year to 3 years
    B. birth to 3 years
    C. birth to 2 years
    D. birth to 1 year

41. In a child who is conscious and choking, the nurse should attempt to relieve the obstruction if the victim:
    A. is making sounds.
    B. has an effective cough.
    C. has stridor.
    D. all of the above

42. Match the drug used for pediatric emergency care with its use during resuscitation.

A. sodium bicarbonate

_____ increases cardiac output and heart rate by blocking vagal stimulation in the heart

B. calcium chloride

_____ antidysrhythmic that is used if lidocaine is ineffective

C. bretylium

_____ used for hypermagnesemia; needed for normal cardiac contractility

D. adenosine

_____ causes vasoconstriction and increases cardiac output

E. dopamine

_____ used for ventricular dysrhythmias

F. lidocaine

_____ acts on alpha- and beta-adrenergic receptor sites, causing contraction especially at the site of the heart, vascular, and other smooth muscle

G. epinephrine

H. atropine

_____ administer rapidly; causes a temporary block through the atrioventricular node

_____ used to buffer the pH

43. The Heimlich maneuver is recommended for children over the age of:
    A. 4 years.
    B. 3 years.
    C. 2 years.
    D. 1 year.

❖ Critical Thinking ❖
Case Study

44. A 14-month-old male child is admitted to the pediatric unit with a respiratory infection. If he has the cough which is characteristic of croup, the nurse would expect to hear:
    A. paroxysmal cough with an inspiratory "whoop."
    B. a brassy cough.
    C. a very severe cough.
    D. a quiet cough.

45. If the child has no cough at all, the nurse would begin to suspect:
    A. cystic fibrosis.
    B. pertussis.
    C. pneumonia.
    D. measles.

46. The child is placed under mist tent with 40% oxygen. Chest physiotherapy and intravenous antibiotics are started. The nurse is monitoring his oxygen saturation with pulse oximetry. The pulse oximeter alarm sounds and the saturation registers 76%. The nurse should begin the assessment with an evaluation for changes in:
    A. behavior.
    B. skin color.
    C. placement of the oximeter sensor.
    D. hemoglobin.

47. If the child is diagnosed as having pneumonia, which one of the following adjunctive techniques would be of NO value?
    A. intravenous antibiotics
    B. the mist tent at 40% oxygen
    C. pulse oximetry
    D. chest physiotherapy

❖ Crossword Puzzle ❖

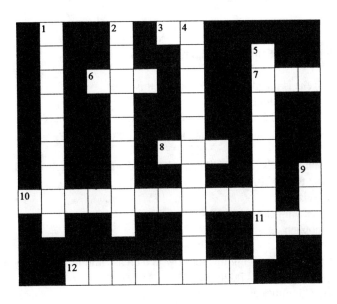

Across

3. Minute volume
6. Cardiopulmonary resuscitation
7. Arterial blood gas
8. Advanced life support
10. Process of oxygen and carbon dioxide exchange within the body
11. Emergency medical services
12. Slow or shallow respirations

Down

1. Deep, rapid, or labored respiration
2. Deficiency of oxygen in the arterial blood
4. Process by which gases are moved into and out of the lungs
5. Abnormally rapid rate of breathing
9. Basic life support

❖ CHAPTER 32
The Child with Respiratory Dysfunction

1. The largest percentage of respiratory infections in children are caused by:
   A. pneumococci.
   B. viruses.
   C. streptococci.
   D. *Haemophilus influenzae.*

2. The MOST likely reason that the respiratory infection rate increases drastically in the age range from 3 to 6 months is that the:
   A. infant's exposure to pathogens is greatly increased during this time.
   B. viral agents that are mild in older children are extremely severe in infants.
   C. maternal antibodies have decreased and the infant's own antibody production is immature.
   D. diameter of the airways is smaller in the infant than in the older child.

3. Which one of the following situations is LEAST likely to be associated with a febrile seizure?
   A. a sudden rise in temperature to 104° F
   B. a family history of febrile seizures
   C. a 6-year-old child develops a temperature of 104° F
   D. administration of acetaminophen

4. The primary concern of the nurse when giving tips for how to increase humidity in the home of a child with a respiratory infection should be to make sure the child has:
   A. continuous contact with the humidification source.
   B. a warm humidification source.
   C. a humidification source that is safe.
   D. all of the above.

5. Which one of the following options would be the BEST choice for the child with a respiratory disorder who needs bedrest but who is not cooperating?
   A. Be sure the mother takes the advice seriously.
   B. Allow the child to play quietly on the floor.
   C. Insist that the child play quietly in bed.
   D. Allow the child to cry until he/she stays in bed.

6. For children who are having difficulty breathing through their noses because of a stuffy nose, the nurse should recommend:
   A. dextromethorphan nose drops.
   B. phenylephrine nose drops.
   C. dextromethorphan cough lozenges.
   D. steroid nose drops.

7. Children with nasopharyngitis may be treated with:
   A. decongestants.
   B. antihistamines.
   C. expectorants.
   D. all of the above.

8. The BEST technique to prevent spread of nasopharyngitis is:
   A. prompt immunization.
   B. to avoid contact with infected persons.
   C. mist vaporization.
   D. to ensure adequate fluid intake.

9. Group A beta-hemolytic streptococcal infection is usually a:
   A. serious infection of the upper airway.
   B. common cause of pharyngitis in children over the age of 15 years.
   C. brief illness that places the child at risk for serious sequelae.
   D. disease of the heart, lungs, joints, and central nervous system.

10. Clinical diagnosis of group A beta-hemolytic streptococcal infection is usually based on:
    A. antibody responses.
    B. antistreptolysin O responses.
    C. complete blood count.
    D. throat culture.

11. Offensive mouth odor, persistent dry cough, and a voice with a muffled nasal quality are commonly the result of:
    A. tonsillectomy.
    B. adenoidectomy.
    C. mouth breathing.
    D. otitis media.

12. Viral tonsillitis is more common than group A beta-hemolytic streptococcus in which one of the following age groups?
    A. 9 to 12 years
    B. 6 to 9 years
    C. 3 to 6 years
    D. 0 to 3 years

13. An adenoidectomy would be CONTRAINDICATED in a child:
    A. with recurrent otitis media.
    B. with malignancy.
    C. with thrombocytopenia.
    D. under the age of 3 years.

14. In the postoperative period following a tonsillectomy, the child should be:
    A. placed in Trendelenburg position.
    B. encouraged to cough and deep breathe.
    C. suctioned vigorously to clear the airway.
    D. placed on bedrest for the day of surgery.

15. Pain medication for the child in the postoperative period following a tonsillectomy should be administered:
    A. orally at regular intervals.
    B. orally as needed.
    C. rectally or intravenously at regular intervals.
    D. rectally or intravenously as needed.

16. Which one of the following foods is MOST appropriate to offer first to an alert child who is in the postoperative period following a tonsillectomy?
    A. ice cream
    B. red gelatin
    C. flavored ice pops
    D. All of the above are appropriate.

17. Which one of the following signs is an early indication of hemorrhage in a child who has had a tonsillectomy?
    A. frequent swallowing
    B. decreasing blood pressure
    C. restlessness
    D. all of the above

18. Which one of the following findings is almost always present in an adolescent with infectious mononucleosis?
    A. skin rash
    B. otitis media
    C. hepatic involvement
    D. failure to thrive

19. Diagnosis of infectious mononucleosis is established when the:
    A. leukocyte count is elevated.
    B. leukocyte count is depressed.
    C. antibody testing is positive.
    D. antibody testing is negative.

20. Infectious mononucleosis is usually a:
    A. disease complicated with pneumonitis and anemia.
    B. self-limiting disease.
    C. disabling disease.
    D. difficult and prolonged disease.

21. Clinical manifestations of influenza would usually include all of the following EXCEPT:
    A. nausea and vomiting.
    B. fever and chills.
    C. sore throat and dry mucous membranes.
    D. photophobia and myalgia.

22. The infant is predisposed to developing otitis media because the eustachian tubes:
    A. lie in a relatively horizontal plane.
    B. have a limited amount of lymphoid tissue.
    C. are long and narrow.
    D. are underdeveloped.

23. List five complications of otitis media.

    _____

    _____

    _____

    _____

    _____

24. The clinical manifestations of otitis media include:
    A. purulent discharge in the external auditory canal.
    B. clear discharge in the external auditory canal.
    C. enlarged axillary lymph nodes.
    D. enlarged cervical lymph nodes.

25. An abnormal otoscopic examination would reveal:
    A. visible landmarks.
    B. a light reflex.
    C. dull gray tympanic membrane.
    D. mobile tympanic membrane.

26. Which one of the following antibiotics would usually be prescribed for otitis media?
    A. tetracycline
    B. amoxicillin
    C. gentamicin
    D. methicillin

27. To help alleviate the discomfort and fever of otitis media, the nurse may administer:
    A. acetaminophen or ibuprofen.
    B. antihistamines and decongestants.
    C. analgesic ear drops.
    D. all of the above.

28. Which one of the following techniques would be CONTRAINDICATED for the nurse to recommend to parents to prevent recurrent otitis externa?
    A. Administer a combination of vinegar and alcohol after swimming.
    B. Allow the child to swim every day.
    C. Dry the ear canal with a cotton swab after swimming.
    D. Use a hair dryer on low heat at 1 to 2 feet for 30 seconds several times a day.

29. Most children with croup syndrome:
    A. require hospitalization.
    B. will need to be intubated.
    C. can be cared for at home.
    D. are over 6 years old.

30. Which one of the following croup syndromes is potentially life-threatening?
    A. spasmodic croup
    B. laryngotracheobronchitis
    C. acute spasmodic laryngitis
    D. epiglottitis

31. The nurse should suspect epiglottitis if the child has:
    A. cough, sore throat, and agitation.
    B. cough, drooling, and retractions.
    C. absence of cough, drooling, and agitation.
    D. absence of cough, hoarseness, and retractions.

32. In the child who is suspected of having epiglottitis, the nurse should:
    A. have intubation equipment available.
    B. prepare to immunize the child for *Haemophilus influenzae*.
    C. obtain a throat culture.
    D. all of the above

33. Since the advent of immunization for *Haemophilus influenzae*, there has been a decrease in the incidence of:
    A. laryngotracheobronchitis.
    B. epiglottitis.
    C. Reye's syndrome.
    D. croup syndrome.

34. Which one of the following children is MOST likely to be hospitalized for treatment of croup?
    A. the 2-year-old child whose croupy cough worsens at night
    B. the 5-year-old child whose croupy cough worsens at night
    C. the 2-year-old child using the accessory muscles to breath
    D. the child with inspiratory stridor during the physical examination

35. Which one of the following choices includes the primary therapeutic regimens for croup?
    A. vigilant assessment, racemic epinephrine, and corticosteroids
    B. vigilant assessment, racemic epinephrine, and antibiotics
    C. intubation, racemic epinephrine, and corticosteroids
    D. intubation, racemic epinephrine, and antibiotics

36. The nurse should expect to intubate the child diagnosed with:
    A. acute spasmodic laryngitis.
    B. bacterial tracheitis.
    C. acute laryngotracheobronchitis.
    D. acute laryngitis.

37. Respiratory syncytial virus is:
    A. an uncommon virus that causes severe bronchiolitis.
    B. an uncommon virus that usually does not require hospitalization.
    C. a common virus that usually causes severe bronchiolitis.
    D. a common virus that usually does not require hospitalization.

38. In the infant who is admitted with possible respiratory syncytial virus, the nurse would expect the lab to perform:
    A. the ELISA antibody test on nasal secretions.
    B. a viral culture of the stool.
    C. a bacterial culture of nasal secretions.
    D. an anaerobic culture of the blood.

39. The use of ribavirin for respiratory syncytial virus is controversial because:
    A. it has been shown to be ineffective.
    B. of the potential toxic effects to health care workers.
    C. it has been shown to be no more effective than antibiotics.
    D. The American Academy of Pediatrics will not endorse its use.

40. Nurses caring for a child with respiratory syncytial virus should:
    A. have a skin test every six months.
    B. wear gloves and gowns when entering the room.
    C. turn off the aerosol machine before opening the tent.
    D. not take care of other children with respiratory syncytial virus at the same time.

41. Match the age of the child with the common cause of pneumonia in that age group.

    A. *Haemophilus influenzae*   _____   over 5 years of age

    B. *Streptococcus pneumoniae*   _____   3 months to 5 years of age

    C. mycoplasmal pneumonia   _____   under 3 months of age

42. Closed chest drainage is MOST likely to be used in:
    A. *Haemophilus pneumoniae.*
    B. mycoplasmal pneumonia.
    C. streptococcal pneumonia.
    D. staphylococcal pneumonia.

43. In an 8-month-old infant admitted to the hospital with pertussis, the nurse should particularly assess the:
    A. living conditions of the infant.
    B. labor and delivery history of the mother.
    C. immunization status of the infant.
    D. alcohol and drug intake of the mother.

44. The BEST test to screen for tuberculosis is the:
    A. chest x-ray.
    B. purified protein derivative (PPD) test.
    C. sputum culture.
    D. multipuncture test (MPT) like the tine test.

45. The child who has active tuberculosis is treated with:
    A. isoniazid.
    B. rifampin.
    C. pyrazinamide.
    D. all of the above.

46. The usual site of bronchial obstruction is the:
    A. left bronchus because it is shorter and straighter.
    B. left bronchus because it is longer and angled.
    C. right bronchus because it is shorter and straighter.
    D. right bronchus because it is longer and angled.

47. The definitive diagnosis of foreign airway bodies in the trachea and larynx is usually made based on:
    A. radiographic examination.
    B. fluoroscopic examination.
    C. bronchoscopic examination.
    D. ultrasonographic examination.

48. Parents may be taught to deal with the aspiration of a foreign body in an infant under 12 months old by using:
    A. back blows and chest thrusts.
    B. back blows only.
    C. the Heimlich maneuver only.
    D. a blind finger sweep.

49. The child who has ingested lighter fluid usually receives:
    A. the same treatment as a child who has hepatitis.
    B. medication to induce vomiting.
    C. the same treatment as a child who has pneumonia.
    D. activated charcoal.

50. List at least five physical findings commonly seen in the child with allergic rhinitis.

    _____

    _____

    _____

    _____

    _____

51. Which one of the following children is most likely suffering from allergy rather than a cold?
    A. a 2-year-old with fever and a runny nose
    B. an adolescent with itchy eyes and constant sneezing without fever
    C. a 2-year-old with sporadic sneezing and a runny nose
    D. an adolescent with sporadic sneezing and a runny nose

❖ Critical Thinking ❖
Case Study

Jason Wilson, who is 8 years old, is admitted to the pediatric unit with the diagnosis of reactive airway disease. This is his first hospitalization for this disorder. Both of Jason's parents smoke cigarettes, but they try to smoke outdoors. Jason usually does quite well. His asthma tends to increase in severity during the winter months. This year he has had several colds and his asthma has flared up each time. This time, however, he is quite uncomfortable. He has audible wheezes in all lung fields.

52. Which one of the following questions would be important for the nurse to ask Jason's mother?
    A. "What brings you to the hospital?"
    B "What is your ethnic background?"
    C. "Do you have a history of asthma in your family?"
    D. "Was your pregnancy and delivery uneventful?"

53. Mrs. Wilson wants the nurse to explain exactly what reactive airway disease means. She says she has been told many times, but it is always when Jason is in so much distress that she is not sure she hears it correctly. The nurse would respond knowing that:
    A. asthma is caused by a certain inflammatory mediator.
    B. the one mechanism responsible for the obstructive symptoms of asthma is excess mucus secretion.
    C. the one mechanism responsible for the obstructive symptoms of asthma is spasm of the smooth muscle of the bronchi.
    D. most theories do not explain all types and causes of asthma.

54. In general, Jason does not have difficulty with any food or emotional triggers for the asthma. An asthmatic episode for Jason starts with itching all over the upper part of his back. He is usually quite irritable and very restless. He complains of headache, chest tightness, and tiredness. He usually will cough, sweat, and sit upright with his shoulders in a hunched-over position. Today he has no fever and is in the tripod position. His skin is sweaty. Based on this information, the nurse would decide that Jason is:
    A. severely ill.
    B. moderately ill.
    C. mildly ill.
    D. not ill at all.

55. Jason's younger sister Tanya is an infant. Tanya's asthma is much worse than Jason's. Mrs. Wilson states that Tanya often has movements of her chest muscles which look as if she is working very hard to breathe, but her respiratory rate does not change. When this is happening Tanya is not breathing a long breath out like Jason does. These differences between Jason and Tanya are confusing to Mrs. Wilson, and she asks the nurse for advice about what to do when this happens to Tanya. The nurse's response is based on the knowledge that:
    A. dyspnea is much more difficult to evaluate in an infant than in a young child.
    B. infant's and young children's bodies respond to the asthmatic episode the same way.
    C. boys tend to have a more severe disease of asthma than girls.
    D. dyspnea is much more difficult to evaluate in a young child than in an infant.

56. The nurse examines Jason and finds that he has hyperresonance on percussion. His breath sounds are coarse and loud with sonorous crackles throughout the lung fields. Expiration is prolonged; rales can be heard. There is generalized inspiratory and expiratory wheezing. Based on these findings, the nurse suspects that there is:
    A. minimal obstruction.
    B. significant obstruction.
    C. imminent ventilatory failure.
    D. an extrathoracic obstruction.

57. The nurse administers a peak flow inspirometer and determines that Jason's peak expiratory flow rate is in the yellow zone. The nurse recognizes that this test result indicates that Jason's asthma control is about:
    A. 80% of his personal best and his routine treatment plan can be followed.
    B. 50% of his personal best and he needs an increase in his usual therapy.
    C. 50% of his personal best and he needs immediate bronchodilators.
    D. less than 50% of his personal best and he needs immediate bronchodilators.

58. Jason's test results are back from the lab. The white blood cell count is $11,200/mm^3$. The eosinophils are $728/mm^3$. The chest x-ray shows infiltrates and hyperexpansion of the airways. The nurse knows that these findings:
    A. support the diagnosis of pneumonia without an episode of asthma.
    B. support the diagnosis of asthma complicated with pneumonia.
    C. do not support the diagnosis of an acute episode of asthma or pneumonia.
    D. support the diagnosis of acute episode of asthma without pneumonia.

59. The physician orders albuterol via inhaler for Jason. Mrs. Wilson is very concerned because she says that Jason usually receives theophylline intravenously. The nurse's response is based on the fact that:
    A. Jason's asthma episode is probably not as severe as usual.
    B. Jason's physician must be using information that is outdated.
    C. theophylline is a third-line drug because it has no more benefit than nebulized beta agonists.
    D. theophylline is a third-line drug because it has been shown to adversely affect school performance.

60. Jason's physician has ordered a corticosteroid via aerosol in addition to the albuterol. Which aerosol medication should the nurse administer first?
    A. albuterol
    B. corticosteroid

61. Based on the nurse's assessment, a care plan is developed. Which one of the following nursing diagnoses would be LEAST likely to appear on Jason's care plan?
    A. activity intolerance related to imbalance between oxygen supply and demand
    B. ineffective airway clearance related to allergenic response and inflammation in the bronchial tree
    C. high risk for infection related to the presence of infective organisms
    D. altered family processes related to a chronic illness

62. When preparing for discharge, the nurse would MOST likely plan to teach the Wilson family to:
    A. keep the humidity at home above 50%.
    B. vacuum the carpets at least twice weekly.
    C. treat carpets with a 3% tannic acid solution.
    D. launder sheets/blankets regularly in cold water.

63. Jason uses aerosolized steroids at home; therefore, he should be taught to rinse his mouth thoroughly with water:
    A. before each treatment to increase absorption.
    B. after each treatment to minimize the risk of oral candidiasis.
    C. before each treatment to minimize the adverse effects of the drug.
    D. after each treatment to increase absorption.

64. Which one of the following principles should be a part of Jason's home self-management program?
   A. Individuals must learn not to abuse their medications so that they will not become addicted.
   B. It is easy to treat an asthmatic episode as long as the child knows the symptoms.
   C. Although quite uncommon, asthma is very treatable.
   D. Children with asthma are usually able to participate in the same activities as nonasthmatic children.

❖ Critical Thinking ❖
Case Study

Andrea MacAuley is an 8-year-old with cystic fibrosis. She is in the fifth percentile for both height and weight. This failure to thrive persists even though she has a voracious appetite. She has been managed at home most recently for about six months without the need for hospitalization. She is admitted today with blood-tinged sputum. The sputum culture obtained two days ago is positive for pseudomonas. The nurse hears rales in both lungs, and Andrea has significant clubbing of her fingers with a capillary refill time of greater than five seconds.

65. Based on the information presented in Andrea MacAuley's case study, the nurse suspects that Andrea's:
   A. condition is improving and she will soon return to home care.
   B. condition is progressively worsening.
   C. condition is worse, but intravenous antibiotic therapy will correct the problem.
   D. family has been noncompliant, causing this setback.

66. The admission orders included an order for gentamicin at a dose that the nurse calculated to be higher than usual for a child of Andrea's size. This dose may be high due to the fact that:
   A. the physician used Andrea's age rather than her size to determine the dose.
   B. the pharmacy has made an error.
   C. children with cystic fibrosis metabolize antibiotics rapidly.
   D. children with cystic fibrosis metabolize antibiotics slowly.

67. Which one of the following strategies would most likely be CONTRAINDICATED for Andrea to use?
   A. forced expiration
   B. aerobic exercise
   C. chest physiotherapy
   D. high-flow oxygen therapy

68. The blood-tinged sputum progresses to an amount greater than 300 cc per day. The nurse recognizes that increased tendency to bleed may be a result of:
   A. iron deficiency anemia.
   B. vitamin K deficiency.
   C. thrombocytopenia.
   D. vitamin D deficiency.

69. Family support for Andrea will most likely include strategies for all of the following issues EXCEPT:
   A. pregnancy and genetic counseling.
   B. relief from the continual routine with respite care.
   C. dealing with a chronic illness and anticipatory grieving.
   D. abnormal psychological adjustment and dysfunctional family patterns.

70. Andrea takes 7 pancreatic enzyme capsules about 30 minutes before each meal. She usually has two to three bowel movements per day. Which one of the following statements is CORRECT in regard to Andrea's pancreatic enzyme dosage?
   A. The dosage is adequate.
   B. The dosage should always be fewer than 5 capsules.
   C. The dosage should be 7 to 10 capsules.
   D. The dosage is adequate, but she should take it after meals.

❖ Crossword Puzzle ❖

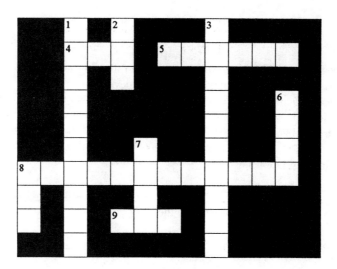

Across

4. Acute otitis media
5. Acute nasal congestion
8. Inflammation of the epiglottis
9. Metered-dose inhaler

Down

1. Inflammation of the larynx
2. Otitis media with effusion
3. Inflammation of the bronchi
6. Adult respiratory distress syndrome
7. Chronic obstructive pulmonary disease
8. Exercise-induced asthma

❖ CHAPTER 33
The Child with Gastrointestinal Dysfunction

1. The functions of the GI system do NOT include which one of the following?
   A. process and absorb nutrients necessary to support growth and development
   B. maintain thermoregulatory functions
   C. perform excretory functions
   D. maintain fluid and electrolyte balance

2. Fill in the blanks in the following statements.

   A. Three processes, _____, _____, and _____, are necessary to convert nutrients into forms that can be utilized by the body.

   B. Chemical digestion involves five general types of GI secretions: _____, _____,

   _____ _____, _____, and _____ ____

   _____.

   C. The _____ _____ is the principal absorption site in the GI system.

   D. The most important nursing assessments included in GI assessment are _____ and

   _____, _____ and _____, _____

   _____, and simple laboratory tests of _____ and _____.

3. The nurse is preparing Dottie, age 7, for an upper GI endoscopy. Which one of the following does the nurse recognize as NOT being an appropriate preparation for this test?
   A. bowel cleansing with magnesium citrate or Golytely
   B. NPO for 8 hours before the procedure
   C. Dottie will need to be given sedation before the procedure is begun.
   D. The nurse will need to explain to Dottie in advance about the procedure by use of pictures or play with dolls and demonstration.

4. Match the term with its description.

A. pica

B. failure to thrive

C. regurgitation

D. projectile vomiting

E. encopresis

F. hematemesis

G. hematochezia

H. melena

I. dysphagia

J. Hemoccult test

K. stool for O & P (ova and parasites)

_____ aids in the diagnosis of parasitic infections

_____ detects presence of blood in the stool

_____ vomiting of bright red blood as a result of bleeding in the upper GI tract or swallowed blood from the upper respiratory tract

_____ passage of bright red blood from the rectum

_____ passage of dark-colored "tarry" stools

_____ difficulty swallowing

_____ eating disorder in which there is compulsive eating of both food and nonfood substances

_____ deceleration from normal pattern of growth or below the 5th percentile

_____ a backward flowing such as return of gastric contents into the mouth

_____ accompanied by vigorous peristaltic waves

_____ outflow of incontinent stool, causing soiling

5. Ben, a 2-year-old, has been brought to the clinic because his parents are afraid he has swallowed a small button battery from his father's watch, which he was playing with. The nurse recognizes which one of the following as the MOST appropriate nursing action at this time?
   A. Reassure the parents that Ben has probably not swallowed the battery because he has no symptoms, he is playing in the examination room, and his lung fields are clear.
   B. Explain to the parents that Ben will probably be allowed to normally pass the battery through the GI system because Ben has been able to eat and drink normally since the event.
   C. Start immediate teaching of Ben's parents on how to assess Ben's environment for hazardous objects and how to assess Ben's toys and other items he might play with for safety.
   D. Explain to Ben's parents that x-ray examination will be conducted, and the battery will probably need to be removed to prevent local damage.

6. The nurse is counseling the mother of 12-month-old Brian on methods to prevent constipation. Which one of the following methods would be CONTRAINDICATED for Brian?
   A. Add bran to Brian's cereal.
   B. Increase Brian's intake of water.
   C. Add prunes to Brian's diet.
   D. Add popcorn to Brian's diet.

7. Sally, age 5, is started on a bowel habit retraining program for chronic constipation. Instructions to the family should include which one of the following?
   A. Decrease the water and increase the milk in Sally's diet.
   B. Establish a regular toilet time twice a day after meals when Sally will sit on the toilet for 5 to 15 minutes.
   C. Withhold Sally's play time with her friend Julie if she does not have a daily bowel movement.
   D. Have Sally sit on the toilet each day until she has a bowel movement.

8. To confirm the diagnosis of Hirschsprung disease, the nurse prepares the child for which one of the following tests?
   A. barium enema
   B. upper GI series
   C. rectal biopsy
   D. esophagoscopy

9. The nurse would expect to see what clinical manifestations in the child diagnosed with Hirschsprung disease?
   A. history of bloody diarrhea, fever, and vomiting
   B. irritability, severe abdominal cramps, and fecal soiling
   C. decreased hemoglobin, increased serum lipids, and positive stool for O & P (ova and parasites)
   D. history of constipation, abdominal distention, and palpable fecal mass

10. The nurse instructs the parents of Gail, a 2-month-old with gastroesophageal reflux, to include which one of the following in Gail's care?
    A. Stop breast-feeding Gail since breast milk is too thin and easily leads to reflux.
    B. After feeding and burping Gail, position her prone with the head and chest elevated 30 degrees.
    C. After feeding and burping Gail, position her on her back with the head turned to the side.
    D. Try to increase feeding volume right before bedtime because this is the time when the stomach is more able to retain foods.

11. The MOST common clinical manifestations expected with Meckel diverticulum include which one of the following?
    A. fever, vomiting, and constipation
    B. weight loss, hypotension, and obstruction
    C. painless rectal bleeding, abdominal pain, or intestinal obstruction
    D. abdominal pain, bloody diarrhea, and foul-smelling stool

12. The child presenting with irritable bowel syndrome is MOST likely to represent which one of the following?
    A. history of colic with feeding difficulties and a family history of bowel problems
    B. alternating patterns of constipation and bloody diarrhea with little flatulence
    C. history of parasitic infections, poor nutrition, and low abdominal pain
    D. history of colic, laxative abuse, and growth retardation

13. Which one of the following would alert the nurse to possible peritonitis from a ruptured appendix in a child suspected of having appendicitis?
    A. colicky abdominal pain with guarding of the abdomen
    B. periumbilical pain that progresses to the lower right quadrant of the abdomen with an elevated WBC
    C. low-grade fever of 100.6° F with the child having difficulty walking and assuming a side-lying position with the knees flexed toward the chest
    D. temperature of 103° F, absent bowel sounds, and sudden relief from abdominal pain

14. A common feature of inflammatory bowel disease is:
    A. growth abnormalities.
    B. chronic constipation.
    C. obstruction.
    D. burning epigastric pain.

15. Nursing considerations for the adolescent with inflammatory bowel disease include:
    A. assisting the adolescent cope with feelings of being different from peers and negative self-esteem.
    B. encouraging three large meals a day of high-protein, high-caloric foods.
    C. stopping drug therapy with remission of symptoms.
    D. elimination of all high-fiber foods from the diet.

16. Which one of the following is NOT thought to contribute to peptic ulcer disease?
    A. *Helicobacter pylori*
    B. alcohol and smoking
    C. caffeine-containing beverages and spicy foods
    D. psychologic factors such as stressful life events

17. Common therapeutic management of peptic ulcer disease includes which one of the following?
    A. corticosteroids
    B. cimetidine or ranitidine
    C. acetaminophen
    D. sulfasalazine and sucralfate

18. Bill, age 1 month, is brought to the clinic by his mother. The nurse suspects pyloric stenosis. Which one of the following symptoms would support this theory?
    A. diarrhea
    B. projectile vomiting
    C. fever and dehydration
    D. abdominal distention

19. Preoperatively, the nursing plan for pyloric obstruction should include which one of the following?
    A. rehydration by intravenous fluids for fluid and electrolyte imbalance
    B. NG tube placement to decompress the stomach
    C. parental support and reassurance
    D. all of the above

20. The single most effective measurement in prevention and control of hepatitis is _____.

21. An invagination of one portion of the intestine into another is called:
    A. intussusception.
    B. pyloric stenosis.
    C. tracheoesophageal fistula.
    D. Hirschsprung disease.

22. Al, age 5 months, is suspected of having intussusception. What clinical manifestations would he MOST likely have?
    A. crying with abdominal examination, vomiting, and currant-jelly-appearing stools
    B. fever, diarrhea, vomiting, and lowered WBC
    C. weight gain, constipation, and refusal to eat
    D. abdominal distention, periodic pain, and hypotension

23. Al's intussusception is reduced during the diagnostic barium enema. The nurse should expect care for Al after the reduction to include:
    A. administration of antibiotics.
    B. enema administration to remove remaining stool.
    C. observation of stools.
    D. rectal temperatures every four hours.

24. The MOST important therapeutic management for the child with celiac disease is:
    A. eliminating corn, rice, and millet from the diet.
    B. adding iron, folic acid, and fat-soluble vitamins to the diet.
    C. eliminating wheat, rye, barley, and oats from the diet.
    D. educating the child's parents about the short-term effects of the disease and the necessity of reading all food labels for content until the disease is in remission.

25. The prognosis for children with short bowel syndrome has improved as a result of:
    A. dietary supplemental vitamin B$_{12}$ additions.
    B. improvement in surgical procedures to correct the deficiency.
    C. improved home care availability.
    D. total parenteral nutrition and enteral feeding.

26. Jerry, a 4-year-old, is brought to the emergency room by his parents, who say he vomited a large amount of bright red blood. Jerry is pale and cool to the touch, with increased respiratory and heart rates. The nurse expects priority care at this time to NOT include:
    A. administration of intravenous fluids, usually normal saline or lactated Ringer's.
    B. blood diagnostic testing for hemoglobin and hematocrit levels.
    C. insertion of an NG tube for ice water lavage.
    D. having suction equipment available.

27. Match the viral hepatitis type with the statement. (Types may be used more than once.)

    A. hepatitis A   _____ most common form of acute viral hepatitis

    B. hepatitis B   _____ immunity by vaccination available

    C. hepatitis C   _____ non-A, non-B with transmission through the fecal-oral route or with contaminated water

    D. hepatitis D
                            _____ spread directly and indirectly by the fecal-oral route
    E. hepatitis E
                            _____ occurs in children already infected with hepatitis B

                            _____ primary cause of post-transfusion hepatitis; often becomes a chronic condition and can cause cirrhosis

                            _____ incubation period 14 to 180 days; average 50 days

28. Sandy, age 2, is brought to the clinic by her mother because a fellow day school toddler has been diagnosed with hepatitis A. Sandy's mother is concerned that Sandy might develop the disease. Which one of the following serum laboratory tests would indicate that Sandy has immunity to hepatitis A?
    A. anti-HAV IgG
    B. anti-HAV IgM
    C. HAsAg
    D. HAcAg

29. Sandy's testing reflects that she has not had hepatitis A. Because her exposure to hepatitis A occurred within the last two weeks, the nurse would expect the physician to order which one of the following for prophylactic administration?
    A. hepatitis B immune globulin
    B. hepatitis B vaccine
    C. standard immune globulin
    D. vaccine for HAV

30. Which one of the following would NOT be expected in the child diagnosed with cirrhosis?
    A. hepatosplenomegaly
    B. elevated liver function tests
    C. decreased ammonia levels
    D. white-colored stools

❖ Critical Thinking ❖
Case Study

Danny, age 17, is a junior in high school. He comes to the clinic with complaints of loss of appetite, constipation, right lower abdominal pain, and slight fever. The nurse suspects appendicitis.

31. It is important for the nurse to assess and include which of the following in Danny's history?
    A. CBC results
    B. description of progression of Danny's abdominal pain
    C. thorough abdominal examination results
    D. urine results

32. Danny should be advised to avoid which of the following until seen by the physician?
    A. all activity
    B. any laxatives
    C. ice to the abdomen
    D. all of the above

33. Danny is admitted to the hospital with a diagnosis of acute appendicitis. The nurse should institute which one of the following independent nursing actions?
    A. Allow clear liquids only.
    B. Start intravenous fluids with antibiotics.
    C. Insert a nasogastric tube and suction.
    D. Monitor closely for progression of symptoms.

34. Danny is now two hours postoperative. During surgery, Danny's appendix was found to have ruptured before surgery. A priority nursing diagnosis at this time would be:
    A. high risk for infection related to rupture.
    B. pain related to inflamed appendix.
    C. altered growth and development related to hospital care.
    D. anxiety related to knowledge deficit regarding disease.

❖ Crossword Puzzle ❖

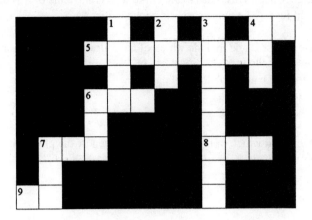

Across

4. Gastrointestinal
5. Yellowish discoloration of the skin and sclera
6. Hepatitis B virus
7. Irritable bowel syndrome
8. Hepatitis A virus
9. Celiac disease; Crohn disease

Down

1. Non-A, non-B virus
2. Chronic nonspecific diarrhea
3. Increased frequency or decreased consistency of stools
4. Gastroesophageal reflux
6. Hypertrophic pyloric stenosis
7. Inflammatory bowel disease

❖ CHAPTER 34
The Child with Cardiovascular Dysfunction

1. The embryologic development of the heart results in a heart beat by the:
   A. fourth week.
   B. fifth week.
   C. sixth week.
   D. eighth week.

2. During the embryologic development of the lower heart, chambers are formed from:
   A. a common ventricle.
   B. the sinus venosus.
   C. a common atrium.
   D. the truncus arteriosus.

3. Part of the process of the formation of the heart's atrial septum results in a temporary flap called the:
   A. truncus arteriosus.
   B. foramen ovale.
   C. sinus venosus.
   D. ductus venosus.

4. In fetal circulation the ductus venosus bypasses the:
   A. heart.
   B. lungs.
   C. liver.
   D. placenta.

5. In fetal circulation the majority of oxygenated blood is pumped through the:
   A. foramen ovale.
   B. lungs.
   C. liver.
   D. coronary sinus.

6. When obtaining a history from the parents of an infant suspected of having altered cardiac function, the nurse would expect to hear:
   A. specific concerns related to the infant's increased activity level.
   B. vague nonspecific complaints such as feeding difficulties.
   C. specific concerns about the infant's shortness of breath.
   D. all of the above.

7. Which disease in the mother during pregnancy is an important clue to the diagnosis of congenital heart disease?
   A. rheumatoid arthritis
   B. rheumatic fever
   C. streptococcal infection
   D. rubella

8. Coarctation of the aorta should be suspected when:
   A. the blood pressure in the arms is different from the blood pressure in the legs.
   B. the blood pressure in the right arm is different from the blood pressure in the left arm.
   C. the apical pulse is greater than the radial pulse.
   D. the point of maximum impulse is shifted to the left.

9. Which one of the following descriptions of heart sounds would be considered normal in a young child?
   A. splitting of S_1
   B. splitting of S_2

10. The standard pediatric electrocardiogram has:
    A. 6 leads.
    B. 12 leads.
    C. 15 leads.
    D. 18 leads.

11. The test that requires intravenous sedation and has been used increasingly in recent years to confirm the diagnosis of a congenital heart defect without a cardiac catheterization is the:
    A. electrocardiogram.
    B. echocardiogram.
    C. transesophageal echocardiogram.
    D. two-dimensional echocardiogram.

12. In children, the usual approach to the left ventricle of the heart in a cardiac catheterization is through the:
    A. left side of the heart.
    B. right side of the heart.

13. List five of the most significant complications following a cardiac catheterization in an infant or young child.

    _____

    _____

    _____

    _____

    _____

14. If bleeding occurs at the insertion site after a cardiac catheterization, the nurse should apply:
    A. warmth to the unaffected extremity.
    B. pressure one inch below the insertion site.
    C. warmth to the affected extremity.
    D. pressure one inch above the insertion site.

15. When children develop congestive heart failure from a congenital heart defect, the failure is usually:
    A. right-sided only.
    B. left-sided only.
    C. cor pulmonale.
    D. both right- and left-sided.

16. Which one of the following heart rates would be tachycardia in an infant?
    A. a resting heart rate of 120 beats per minute
    B. a crying heart rate of 200 beats per minute
    C. a resting heart rate of 160 beats per minute
    D. a crying heart rate of 180 beats per minute

17. Labored breathing in an infant may be identified by:
    A. inability to feed.
    B. circumoral cyanosis.
    C. costal retractions.
    D. all of the above.

18. Developmental delays in the infant with congestive heart failure are MOST pronounced in the:
    A. fine motor areas.
    B. gross motor areas.
    C. social skill areas.
    D. cognitive areas.

19. Evaluation of the infant for edema is different from the older child in that:
    A. weight is not reliable as an early sign.
    B. pedal edema will be most pronounced in the newborn.
    C. edema is usually generalized and difficult to detect.
    D. distended neck veins are the most reliable sign.

20. In the child taking digoxin, electrocardiographic signs that the drug is having the intended effect are:
    A. prolonged PR interval and slowed ventricular rate.
    B. shortened PR interval and slowed ventricular rate.
    C. prolonged PR interval and faster ventricular rate.
    D. shortened PR interval and faster ventricular rate.

21. The two main angiotensin-converting enzyme (ACE) inhibitors MOST commonly used for children with congestive heart failure are:
    A. digoxin and captopril.
    B. enalapril and captopril.
    C. enalapril and furosemide.
    D. spironolactone and captopril.

22. The electrolyte usually depleted with diuretic therapy is:
    A. sodium.
    B. chloride.
    C. potassium.
    D. magnesium.

23. The nutritional needs of the infant with congestive heart failure are usually:
    A. the same as an adult's.
    B. less than a healthy infant's.
    C. the same as a healthy infant's.
    D. greater than a healthy infant's.

24. The calories are usually increased for an infant with congestive heart failure by:
    A. increasing the number of feedings.
    B. introducing solids into the diet.
    C. increasing the caloric density of the formula.
    D. gavage feeding.

25. Which one of the following clinical manifestations is a sign of chronic hypoxemia?
    A. squatting
    B. polycythemia
    C. clubbing
    D. all of the above

26. Prostaglandin is administered to the newborn with a congenital heart defect to:
    A. close the patent ductus arteriosus.
    B. keep the ductus arteriosus open.
    C. keep the foramen ovale open.
    D. close the foramen ovale.

27. Dehydration must be prevented in children who are hypoxemic because dehydration places the child at risk for:
    A. infection.
    B. cerebral vascular accident.
    C. fever.
    D. air embolism.

28. It would be considered unusual if the parents of a child with a congenital heart defect felt:
    A. self-confident with their parenting abilities.
    B. exhausted and discouraged.
    C. they could not leave their child with anyone.
    D. a fear that the child might die.

29. Match the type of defect with the specific disorder. (Defects may be used more than once.)

    A. defects with decreased pulmonary blood flow   _____ patent ductus arteriosus

    B. mixed defects   _____ coarctation of the aorta

    C. defects with increased pulmonary blood flow   _____ ventricular septal defect

    D. obstructive defects   _____ subvalvular aortic stenosis

                                                            _____ hypoplastic left heart syndrome

                                                            _____ atrioventricular canal defect

                                                            _____ pulmonic stenosis

                                                            _____ tetralogy of Fallot

                                                            _____ aortic stenosis

                                                            _____ tricuspid atresia

                                                            _____ valvular aortic stenosis

                                                            _____ truncus arteriosus

                                                            _____ atrial septal defect

                                                            _____ transposition of the great vessels

30. Which one of the following congenital heart defects has the BEST prognosis?
    A. tetralogy of Fallot
    B. ventricular septal defect
    C. atrial septal defect
    D. hypoplastic left heart syndrome

31. Which of the following defects has the WORST prognosis?
    A. tetralogy of Fallot
    B. atrial ventricular canal defect
    C. transposition of the great vessels
    D. hypoplastic left heart syndrome

32. Which one of the following sets of assessment findings are the MOST frequent clinical manifestations of a congenital heart disorder in an infant or child?
    A. decreased cardiac output and low blood pressure
    B. congestive heart failure and a murmur
    C. increased blood pressure and pulse
    D. dyspnea and bradycardia

33. Surgical intervention is always necessary in the first year of life when an infant is born with:
    A. atrial septal defect.
    B. ventricular septal defect.
    C. transposition of the great vessels.
    D. patent ductus arteriosus.

34. The BEST approach for the nurse to use in regard to discipline for the child with a congenital defect is to:
    A. provide the parents with anticipatory guidance.
    B. teach the parents to overcompensate.
    C. help the parents focus on the child's defect.
    D. teach the parents to use benevolent overreaction.

35. Parents of the child with a congenital heart defect are primarily interested in information about the:
    A. anatomy and physiology of the heart.
    B. pathophysiology and morbidity of the disorder.
    C. prognosis and surgical correction of the disorder.
    D. all of the above

36. Parents of the child with a congenital heart defect should know the signs of congestive heart failure, which include:
    A. poor feeding.
    B. sudden weight gain.
    C. increased efforts to breathe.
    D. all of the above.

37. List three major categories that should be included in a teaching plan for parents of a child with a congenital heart disorder.

    _____

    _____

    _____

38. A visit to the intensive care unit prior to open heart surgery should take place:
    A. several days before the surgery.
    B. at a busy time with a lot to see and hear.
    C. the day before surgery.
    D. several weeks before the surgery.

39. Children who will undergo cardiac surgery should be informed about:
    A. the location of the intravenous lines.
    B. the pain at the intravenous insertion sites.
    C. the need to lie still after surgery.
    D. all of the above.

40. Which one of the following patterns is indicative of infection in the postoperative period following cardiac surgery?
    A. temperature of 38.6° C (101.5° F) 72 hours after surgery
    B. temperature of 37.7° C (100° F) 36 hours after surgery
    C. hypothermia in the early postoperative period
    D. restlessness, agitation, and increased WBC count

41. Following cardiac surgery in a child, congestive heart failure would be suspected if the central venous pressure (CVP) catheter readings began to:
    A. fall with a rise in blood pressure.
    B. rise with a rise in blood pressure.
    C. fall with a fall in blood pressure.
    D. rise with a fall in blood pressure.

42. While suctioning an infant after cardiac surgery, the nurse should:
    A. hyperoxygenate before suctioning.
    B. suction for no more than five seconds.
    C. provide supplemental O_2.
    D. all of the above

43. List five observations the nurse should make while suctioning an infant after cardiac surgery.

    _____

    _____

    _____

    _____

    _____

44. Which one of the following is NOT a common reason for chest tube drainage in the child following cardiac surgery?
    A. removal of secretions
    B. removal of air
    C. prevention of pneumothorax
    D. removal of an empyema

45. Which one of the following strategies is NOT acceptable to include in the care of the child prior to removing chest tube(s) after cardiac surgery?
    A. Explain that the removal is uncomfortable but not painful.
    B. Administer intravenous fentanyl.
    C. Administer intravenous morphine sulfate.
    D. Use a topical anesthetic on the site.

46. The MOST painful part of cardiac surgery for the child is usually the:
    A. thoracotomy incision site.
    B. graft site on the leg.
    C. sternotomy incision site.
    D. intravenous insertion sites.

47. An infant who weighs 7 kg has just returned to the intensive care unit following cardiac surgery. The chest tube has drained 30 cc in the past hour. In this situation, what is the first action for the nurse to take?
    A. Notify the surgeon.
    B. Identify any other signs of hemorrhage.
    C. Suction the patient.
    D. Identify any other signs of renal failure.

48. An infant who weighs 7 kg has just returned to the intensive care unit following cardiac surgery. The urine output has been 20 ml in the past hour. In this situation, what is the first action for the nurse to take?
    A. Notify the surgeon.
    B. Identify any other signs of hypervolemia.
    C. Suction the patient.
    D. Identify any other signs of renal failure.

49. Following cardiac surgery, fluid intake calculations for a child would include:
    A. intravenous fluids.
    B. arterial and CVP line flushes.
    C. fluid used to dilute medications.
    D. all of the above.

50. Following cardiac surgery, fluid output calculations in a child would include:
    A. nasogastric secretions.
    B. blood drawn for analysis.
    C. chest tube drainage.
    D. all of the above.

51. One of the factors that increases blood volume in open heart surgery in children is the postoperative:
    A. reabsorption of potassium.
    B. secretion of antidiuretic hormone.
    C. inhibition of aldosterone.
    D. diffusion of fluid into the interstitial spaces.

52. One of the strategies the nurse can use to progressively increase a child's activity in the period after cardiac surgery is to plan:
    A. to expect some degree of dyspnea.
    B. to ambulate on the first day.
    C. to ambulate after analgesic medication.
    D. all of the above

53. List at least five complications of cardiac surgery in children.

    _____

    _____

    _____

    _____

    _____

54. Techniques to provide emotional support to the child and family following cardiac surgery include:
    A. realizing that some procedures are too difficult for the child to perform.
    B. encouraging the child to be brave.
    C. reassuring the parents that a child's anger or rejection of them is normal.
    D. all of the above.

55. Which one of the following patients with bacterial endocarditis (BE) is at highest risk for mortality?
    A. a 15-year-old with BE caused by bacteria that is susceptible to ampicillin
    B. a 2-month-old infant with no cardiac problems
    C. a 5-year-old child with BE following a mitral valve replacement
    D. a 9-year-old with BE and aortic stenosis

56. One of the MOST important factors in preventing bacterial endocarditis is:
    A. administration of prophylactic antibiotic therapy.
    B. surgical repair of the defect.
    C. administration of prostaglandin to maintain patent ductus arteriosus.
    D. administration of antibiotics after dental work.

57. One of the MOST common findings on physical examination of the child with acute rheumatic heart disease is:
    A. a systolic murmur.
    B. pleural friction rub.
    C. an ejection click.
    D. a split S_2.

58. The test that provides the MOST reliable evidence of recent streptococcal infection is the:
    A. throat culture.
    B. Mantoux test.
    C. elevation of liver enzymes.
    D. antistreptolysin O test.

59. Children who have been treated for rheumatic fever:
    A. do not need additional prophylaxis against bacterial endocarditis.
    B. are immune to rheumatic fever for the rest of their lives.
    C. will have transitory manifestations of chorea for the rest of their lives.
    D. may need antibiotic therapy for years.

60. The peak age for the incidence of Kawasaki disease is in the:
    A. infant age group.
    B. toddler age group.
    C. school-age group.
    D. adolescent age group.

61. Which one of the following doses of aspirin would be considered adequate for the initial treatment of Kawasaki disease for a child who weighs 20 kg?
    A. 80 mg every 6 hours
    B. 100 mg every 6 hours
    C. 500 mg every 6 hours
    D. 2000 mg every 6 hours

62. Kawasaki disease is treated with:
    A. aspirin and gamma globulin.
    B. aspirin and cryoprecipitate.
    C. meperidine hydrochloride and gamma globulin.
    D. meperidine hydrochloride and cryoprecipitate.

63. Because of the drug used for long-term therapy, children with Kawasaki disease are at risk for:
    A. chicken pox.
    B. influenza.
    C. Reye's syndrome.
    D. myocardial infarction.

64. Most cases of hypertension in children are a result of:
    A. essential hypertension.
    B. secondary hypertension.
    C. primary hypertension.
    D. congenital heart defects.

65. Most children with hypertension are managed with:
    A. diuretics.
    B. calcium channel blockers.
    C. treatment of the underlying disease.
    D. all of the above.

66. The nurse's role in relation to hypertension may include:
    A. routine accurate assessment of blood pressure in infants and children.
    B. providing information.
    C. follow-up of the child with hypertension.
    D. all of the above.

67. Elevated cholesterol in childhood:
    A. can predict the long-term risk of heart disease for the individual.
    B. can predict the risk of hypertension in adulthood.
    C. is a major predictor of the adult cholesterol level.
    D. is usually symptomatic.

68. The National Cholesterol Education Program recommends screening for cholesterol in:
    A. children over 5 years of age.
    B. children with a family history of premature cardiovascular disease.
    C. children with congenital heart disease.
    D. all children.

69. Which one of the following disorders is a vasculitis that follows an upper respiratory tract infection?
    A. idiopathic thrombocytopenia
    B. Kaposi sarcoma
    C. Kawasaki disease
    D. Henoch-Schonlein purpura

70. The MOST common kind of cardiomyopathy found in children is:
    A. dilated cardiomyopathy.
    B. hypertrophic cardiomyopathy.
    C. restrictive cardiomyopathy.
    D. secondary cardiomyopathy.

71. The heart transplant procedure that is used MOST often in children is the:
    A. heterotopic heart transplantation.
    B. orthotopic heart transplantation.

❖ Critical Thinking ❖
Case Study

Pauline Smith is a 3-year-old child admitted for repair of an atrial septal defect. Her parents have known about the defect since her birth. She has had numerous respiratory infections with occasional episodes of congestive heart failure in the past year. Pauline has taken digoxin and furosemide in the past but currently takes only vitamins with iron. Her parents state that they are anxious to have the surgery over with so that they can treat Pauline like the other children. They have three other children who are older than Pauline.

72. On admission Pauline is afebrile and playful and has no signs of congestive heart failure. As part of the admission process, the nurse would want to be sure to have a baseline assessment of Pauline's:
    A. sucking and swallowing abilities.
    B. reading ability.
    C. exercise tolerance level.
    D. all of the above

73. When developing a nursing care plan for Pauline, the nurse would MOST likely have identified a nursing diagnosis of:
    A. altered family processes.
    B. ineffective breathing pattern.

74. One of the BEST ways to evaluate whether Pauline and her parents understand the instructions related to preparation for the surgery would be for the nurse to:
    A. review the concepts and draw pictures.
    B. observe the parents as they practice postoperative techniques.
    C. use a doll to demonstrate postoperative techniques to Pauline.
    D. make a home visit after surgery.

❖ Crossword Puzzle ❖

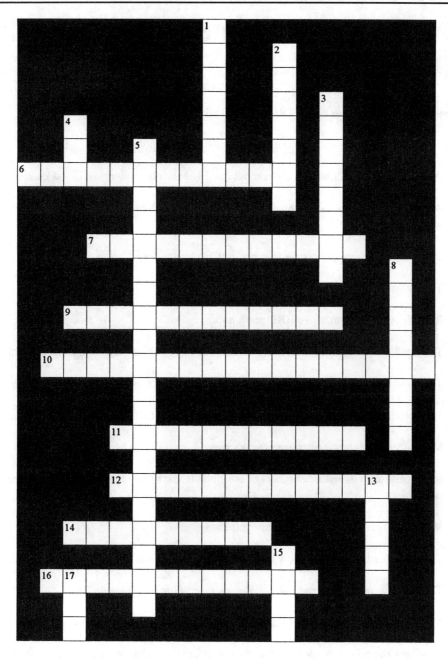

Across

6. Increased number of red blood cells
7. Enlargement of heart muscle
9. Volume of blood ejected by heart during one contraction (2 words)
10. Circulation of blood to tissues throughout body (2 words)
11. Pertaining to movements involved in circulation of blood
12. Ability of heart muscle to pump
14. Pressure that heart must pump against
16. Sequential contraction of heart chambers (2 words)

Down

1. Period of contraction of heart
2. Circulating blood volume returning to heart
3. Period of dilatation of heart
4. Low-density lipoprotein
5. Elevated level of serum cholesterol
8. Bluish color in skin from reduced oxygenation
13. Total anomalous pulmonary venous connection
15. Hypoplastic left heart syndrome
17. Angiotensin-converting enzyme

❖ CHAPTER 35
The Child with Hematologic or Immunologic Dysfunction

1. Identify the following statements as either TRUE or FALSE.

_____ The major physiologic component of red cells is erythropoietin.

_____ A complete blood count with differential describes the components of blood known as platelets.

_____ A child with a suspected bacterial infection would have a differential count that shows a shift to the left with more mature cells present.

_____ Erythrocytes supply oxygen to and remove CO_2 from cells.

_____ The mature RBC has no nucleus.

_____ Reticulocytes indicate active RBC production.

_____ The regulator of erythrocyte production is tissue oxygenation and renal production of erythropoietin.

_____ The regulatory mechanism for the production of erythrocytes is their circulating numbers.

_____ The absolute neutrophil count reflects the body's ability to handle bacterial infection.

_____ Monocytes and lymphocytes are granulocytes.

_____ In the child with increased numbers of eosinophils, the nurse should suspect allergies or parasite infection.

_____ Monocytosis is more evident in acute inflammation.

_____ The hematocrit is approximately three times the hemoglobin content.

_____ The mean corpuscular hemoglobin is the average volume of a single RBC.

_____ Mean corpuscular hemoglobin concentration is the average concentration of hemoglobin in a single cell.

_____ Bands are the immature neutrophils, and they increase in number during bacterial infections.

2. Match the term with its description.

A. normocytes   _____ globular-shaped cells

B. macrocytes   _____ reduced amount of hemoglobin concentration

C. microcytes   _____ sickle-shaped cells

D. spherocytes   _____ sufficient or normal hemoglobin concentration

E. poikilocytes   _____ irregular-shaped cells

F. drepanocytes   _____ normal cell size

G. normochromic   _____ larger than normal cell size

H. hypochromic   _____ smaller than normal cell size

3. The nurse would expect laboratory results for the patient with chronic blood loss to include:
   A. high iron levels.
   B. macrocytic and hyperchromic erythrocytes.
   C. microcytic and hypochromic erythrocytes.
   D. normocytic and normochromic erythrocytes.

4. The most common childhood anemia is _____ _____.

5. Which one of the following is NOT identified as a nurse's role in the treatment of anemia in the pediatric client?
   A. Prepare the child for laboratory tests.
   B. Diagnose complications of therapy.
   C. Decrease tissue oxygen needs.
   D. Implement safety precautions.

6. The nurse is scheduled to administer 100 cc of packed red blood cells to 3-year-old Amy. Which one of the following is NOT a correct guideline when administering the blood?
   A. Take vital signs before administration.
   B. Infuse the blood through an appropriate filter.
   C. Administer 50 cc of the blood within the first few minutes to detect for possible reactions before proceeding with the remainder of the infusion.
   D. Start the blood within 30 minutes of its arrival from the blood bank or return it to the blood bank.

7. Ben, age 7 years, is receiving a transfusion of packed red blood cells. After 45 minutes, he begins to have chills, fever, a sensation of tightness in his chest, and headache. The priority action of the nurse is to:
   A. stop the transfusion and administer acetaminophen.
   B. stop the transfusion and notify the practitioner.
   C. slow the transfusion rate until the symptoms subside.
   D. slow the transfusion and send a sample of the patient's blood and urine to the laboratory for presence of hemo-globin.

8. At birth the normal full-term newborn has maternal stores of iron sufficient to last how long?
   A. the first 5 to 6 months of life
   B. the first 2 to 3 months of life
   C. the first 8 months of life
   D. less than 1 month of life

9. Which one of the following laboratory values is diagnostic of anemia caused by inadequate intake or absorption of iron?
   A. elevated TIBC and reduced SIC
   B. reduced TIBC and SIC
   C. elevated TIBC and SIC
   D. reduced TIBC and elevated SIC

10. Angie, age 11 months, is brought into the clinic by her mother for a routine checkup. On physical examination, the nurse observes that Angie appears chubby, that her skin looks pale and almost porcelain-like, and that Angie has poor muscle development. Based on these observations, which one of the following questions is MOST important for the nurse to include when completing Angie's history?
    A. "Did you have any complications during pregnancy or delivery of Angie?"
    B. "Tell me about what you are currently feeding Angie."
    C. "Has Angie had any recent infections or high fevers?"
    D. "Have you noticed if Angie is having difficulty with her movements or advancing in her growth and development abilities?"

11. The nurse is instructing a new mother in how to prevent iron deficiency anemia in her new premature infant when she takes her home. The mother intends to breast-feed. Which one of the following statements reflects a need for further education of the new mother?
    A. "I will use only breast milk or formula as a source of milk for my baby until she is at least 12 months old."
    B. "My baby will need to have iron supplements introduced when she is 2 months old."
    C. "As my baby is able to tolerate other foods, such as cereal, I should limit her formula intake to about 1 L/day to encourage intake of iron-rich cereals."
    D. "I will need to add iron supplements to my baby's diet when she is 6 months old."

12. When teaching the parents of 4-year-old Tony how to administer the iron supplement ordered for his iron deficiency, the nurse does NOT include which one of the following in the teaching plan?
    A. Give the iron 2 times daily in divided doses with milk.
    B. Give the iron twice daily with orange juice.
    C. Administer the oral liquid iron preparation through a straw to prevent staining of the teeth.
    D. Watch Tony's stools; they will turn a tarry green color and he may become constipated from the iron preparation.

13. Sally and David Brown are returning with Jason, their 6-week-old infant, for a routine newborn examination. Sally is a carrier for sickle cell anemia; David is not. What are the chances that Jason was born with sickle cell anemia?
    A. 25% chance
    B. 50% chance
    C. 75% chance
    D. 0% chance

14. Under conditions of _____, _____, _____, and

    _____ _____, the relatively insoluble HbS changes its molecular structure to filamentous crystals that cause distortion of the cell membrane to a sickle-shaped RBC.

15. Bruce, age 12 years, is admitted to your unit with a diagnosis of sickle cell crisis. Which one of the following activities is MOST likely to have precipitated this episode?
    A. attending the football game with his friends
    B. going camping and hiking in the mountains with his friends
    C. going to the beach and surfing with his friends
    D. staying indoors and reading for several hours

16. Amy is a 5-year-old being admitted because of dimini...
    of sickle cell crisis is she MOST likely experiencing?
    A. vaso-occlusive crisis
    B. splenic sequestration crisis
    C. aplastic crisis
    D. hyperhemolytic crisis

17. Therapeutic management of sickle cell crisis generally incl...
    A. long-term oxygen use to enable the oxygen to reach the s...
    B. increase in activity to promote circulation in the affected ...
    C. diet high in iron to decrease anemia
    D. hydration for hemodilution through oral and IV therapy

18. In controlling pain related to vaso-occlusive sickle cell crisis, w...
    included in the plan of care?
    A. administration of long-term oxygen
    B. application of cold compresses to the area
    C. meperidine (Demerol) to be titrated and administered to a thera...
    D. adding codeine to acetaminophen or ibuprofen if neither one of ... ... in relieving the pain

23. Which one of the following is no longer recom...
    HIV cannot be safely eliminated...
    hepatitis or factor VIII concentrate
    A. cryoprecipitate
    B. DDAVP (1-deamino-8-D-ar...
    C. epsilon aminocaproic aci...
    D. ...

24. Donald, age 5 and p...
    that which of the...
    1. ice packs...
    2. applic...
    3. ad...
    4...

19. Norma, age 2 years, is to begin therapy for beta-thalassemia. Which of the following would be appropriate for the nurse to include in the educational session held with the parents?
    A. Norma will need frequent blood transfusions to keep her Hgb level above 10 g/dl.
    B. To minimize the effect of iron overload, deferoxamine (Desferal), an iron-chelating agent, will be given intravenously or subcutaneously to Norma.
    C. creative strategies to assist the child and parents in complying with the deferoxamine regimen
    D. all of the above

20. Acquired aplastic anemia presents with clinical manifestations of _____, _____,

    and _____ _____ _____.

21. Danny is scheduled to receive antithymocyte globulin (ATG) for treatment of aplastic anemia. Based on knowledge about this therapy, which of the following would the nurse expect?
    A. to watch the intravenous infusion carefully to prevent extravasation of ATG
    B. that the ATG will be given through a central vein
    C. to plan for possible anaphylactic reactions to ATG by having oxygen and epinephrine readily available
    D. all of the above

22. Match the laboratory test for hemostasis with its description.

    A. bleeding time

    B. prothrombin time (PT)

    C. partial thromboplastin time (PTT)

    D. thromboplastin generation test (TGT)

    E. fibrinogen level

    F. hemophilia A

    G. hemophilia B

    _____ allows for determination of specific factor deficiencies, especially factors VIII and IX

    _____ directly measures fibrinogen level in blood

    _____ function depends on platelet aggregation and vasoconstriction

    _____ measures factors necessary for prothrombin conversion to thrombin and fibrogen

    _____ measures the activity of thromboplastin and specific for factor deficiencies except factor VII

    _____ factor IX deficiency

    _____ factor VIII deficiency

...mended for use in treating factor VIII deficiency because the risk of
...?

...inine vasopressin)
...(Amicar, EACA)

...eviously diagnosed with hemophilia A, is being admitted with hemarthrosis. The nurse knows
...following is CONTRAINDICATED in the plan of care for Donald?
...o the affected area
...tion of a splint or sling to the area
...ninistration of corticosteroids
    administration of aspirin, Indocin, or Butazolidin
5. passive range-of-motion exercises
6. active range-of-motion exercises
7. teaching Donald how to administer AHF to himself
A. 1, 3, and 6
B. 2, 3, 4, and 6
C. 1, 5, and 7
D. 4, 5, and 7

25. Which one of the following statements about von Willebrand disease is TRUE?
A. The characteristic clinical feature is an increased tendency toward bleeding from mucous membranes.
B. It affects females but not males.
C. It will be unsafe for the female affected with the disease to have children because of hemorrhage.
D. It is an inherited autosomal recessive disease.

26. An acquired hemorrhagic disorder characterized by excessive destruction of platelets and a discoloration caused by

petechiae beneath the skin is called _____ _____ _____.

27. In severe cases of disseminated intravascular coagulation, treatment may include the administration of heparin. What is the rationale for this therapy?
A. inhibit thrombin formation
B. decrease the platelet count
C. increase the bleeding time
D. all of the above

28. Johnny, age 4 years, comes to the ambulatory outpatient clinic with his mother because she is concerned about a nose-bleed Johnny had this morning. There is no bleeding now, and Johnny's mother reports the nosebleed stopped after about 5 to 10 minutes of direct pressure to the nose area. It was the first nosebleed Johnny has ever had. Examination reflects some old crusted blood located near the anterior part of the nasal septum and what appears as a small scratch in this area. Which one of the following would the nurse expect NOT to be included in the teaching plan for Johnny and his mother?
A. Johnny may have caused the nosebleed by nose picking; he should be encouraged to keep fingers away.
B. Placing a small amount of petroleum or water-soluble jelly inside the nares will lessen the formation of crusting from blood.
C. This nosebleed probably signals an underlying disease process, and Johnny will need full evaluation to eliminate clotting factor deficiency diseases or other abnormalities.
D. Since the nose is a very vascular structure, discourage Johnny from blowing his nose today to decrease the likeli-hood of restarting the bleeding.

29. In child and adolescent age groups, HIV is likely to be transmitted by which of the following methods?
    A. children exposed in utero to an infected mother, or an infected mother may transmit the virus in breast milk
    B. children who received blood products for hemophilia before 1985
    C. adolescents engaged in high-risk behaviors (sexual/drug-related)
    D. all of the above

30. Immunization needs of the child with HIV infection include which one of the following?
    A. delay of all immunizations until the child has the HIV infection under control
    B. not administering pneumococcal and influenza vaccines
    C. using inactivated poliovirus rather than oral poliovirus
    D. varicella zoster immune globulin within one week after exposure to chickenpox

31. Nursing strategies to improve the growth and development of the child with HIV infection should include which one of the following?
    A. Provide high-fat and high-calorie meals and snacks to meet body requirements for growth.
    B. Provide only those foods that the child feels like eating.
    C. Fortify foods with nutritional supplements to maximize quality of intake.
    D. Weigh the child and measure height and muscle mass on a daily basis.

32. Nursing strategies to improve school and peer interactions of the child with HIV infection would BEST include which one of the following?
    A. Encourage the child to have one best friend to whom he/she relates.
    B. Assist the child in identifying personal strengths to facilitate coping.
    C. Tell the child that the hospitalization will not contribute to isolation from peers, and allow the child's friends to send letters.
    D. Discourage the child's parents from allowing school friends to visit the child at home recuperating because rest is especially important for the HIV-infected child.

33. Early clinical manifestations of severe combined immunodeficiency include:
    A. failure to thrive.
    B. delayed developmental milestone achievement.
    C. feeding problems.
    D. susceptibility to infections.

34. In Wiskott-Aldrich syndrome, the MOST notable effect of the disease at birth is which one of the following?
    A. bleeding
    B. infection
    C. eczema
    D. malignancy

❖ Critical Thinking ❖
Case Study

Mary, age 9, has sickle cell anemia. She is admitted to the hospital with knee and back pain and is diagnosed as being in vaso-occlusive crisis.

35. The nurse, in developing a plan of care for Mary, formulated a diagnosis of pain. The nurse understands that Mary's pain is related to which one of the following?
    A. pooling of large amounts of blood in the liver and spleen
    B. shorter life span of the RBCs and the fact that the bone marrow cannot produce enough RBCs
    C. tissue anoxia brought on by sickle cells occluding blood vessels
    D. RBC destruction related to a viral infection or transfusion reaction

36. The nurse is developing an educational plan about sickle cell anemia for Mary and her parents. In order to prevent recurrence of this type of crisis, which one of the following is MOST important to include in the educational session?
   A. Explain the signs of dehydration.
   B. Explain that frequent rest periods are required when the child is in a low-oxygen atmosphere.
   C. Explain that the child should avoid injury to joints to decrease sickling of blood cells.
   D. Explain the importance of avoiding infection by routine immunization and of protection from known sources of infection.

37. Mary is to receive IV fluids to improve hydration. Based on Mary's weight of 60 pounds, the nurse would calculate her minimum fluid requirements per day to be approximately:
   A. 4 liters per day.
   B. 2 liters per day.
   C. 6 liters per day.
   D. 8 liters per day.

38. Evaluation of Mary's progress is BEST based on which one of the following observations?
   A. Mary's verbalization that she no longer has pain or need for pain medication
   B. Mary's ability to perform active range-of-motion exercises
   C. Mary's desire to drink the required level of fluids for hydration
   D. Mary's verbalization of how to prevent future sickle cell crisis

❖ Crossword Puzzle ❖

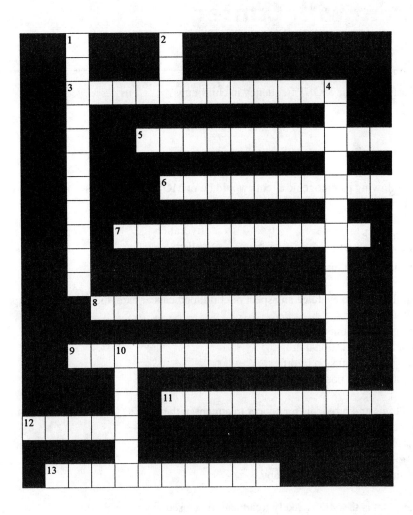

Across

3. Immature RBC
5. One of the major groups of WBCs
6. Granular leukocyte
7. Process of clotting
8. Red blood cell
9. Process of ingesting and digesting foreign proteins
11. Process whereby bleeding from an injured vessel is stopped
12. Remaining plasma after coagulation has taken place
13. Percent of RBCs in total blood volume

Down

1. Platelet
2. Disseminated intravascular coagulation
4. Process of RBC manufacture
10. Reduction of red blood cells or hemoglobin concentration below normal

❖ CHAPTER 36
The Child with Cancer

1. The cancer that occurs with the MOST frequency in children is:
   A. lymphoma.
   B. neuroblastoma.
   C. leukemia.
   D. melanoma.

2. Which one of the following carcinogenic agents would be of MOST concern when considering the development of cancer in children?
   A. low doses of radiation
   B. excessive sun exposure
   C. exposure to cigarette smoke
   D. intramuscular vitamin K at birth

3. When a clinical trial is used to evaluate an aspect of childhood cancer care, the parents can expect that treatment the child receives will always be:
   A. better than the current treatment usually used.
   B. an evaluation of an investigational drug.
   C. intermittent intravenous infusion of drugs.
   D. at least as good as the best possible treatment presently known.

4. The use of clinical trials and protocols for cancer treatment in the past 20 years has resulted in an increased use of:
   A. intermittent intravenous therapy.
   B. continuous intravenous therapy.
   C. lower doses of single-drug therapy.
   D. prolonged duration of maintenance therapy.

5. Bone marrow transplant is the MOST likely treatment to be used when the child:
   A. is unlikely to be cured by other means.
   B. has acute leukemia.
   C. has chronic leukemia.
   D. has a compatible donor in his/her family.

6. Which one of the following children would be MOST likely to develop a malignancy as a result of cancer treatment?
   A. a 18-year-old who receives radiation for treatment of Hodgkin disease
   B. a 2-year-old who receives intrathecal chemotherapy
   C. a 4-year-old who receives radiation for treatment of leukemia
   D. a 15-year-old who receives intrathecal chemotherapy

7. Dental care for a child whose platelet count is $32,000/mm^3$ and granulocyte count is $450/mm^3$ should include:
   A. toothbrushing with flossing.
   B. toothbrushing without flossing.
   C. flossing without toothbrushing.
   D. wiping with moistened sponges.

8. The siblings and household contacts of an immunocompromised child should NOT receive:
   A. any vaccines.
   B. any live attenuated vaccines.
   C. the routine poliovirus vaccine.
   D. live measles, mumps, and rubella (MMR) vaccine.

9. After a bone marrow aspiration is performed on a child, the nurse should:
   A. apply an adhesive bandage.
   B. place the child in Trendelenburg position.
   C. ask the child to remain in the supine position.
   D. apply a pressure bandage.

10. A child who is anemic from myelosuppression should:
    A. strictly limit activities.
    B. regulate his/her own activity with adult supervision.
    C. receive blood transfusions until the hemoglobin level reaches 10.
    D. receive chemotherapy until the hemoglobin level reaches 10.

11. The nursing intervention that would be MOST helpful to use for the child who has stomatitis from cancer chemotherapy would be:
    A. a nonprescription anesthetic preparation without alcohol.
    B. viscous Xylocaine.
    C. lemon glycerin swabs.
    D. Milk of Magnesia.

12. The child who receives reinduction therapy for a relapse in cancer is likely to experience:
    A. more severe alopecia than during the first chemotherapy experience.
    B. thinning of the hair that can leave the hair full enough to make a wig unnecessary.
    C. hair regrowth that is thinner, straighter, and darker than before.
    D. complete baldness, requiring some protection from the cold and sun.

13. Children who develop moon face from steroids used to treat cancer take on an appearance of:
    A. an anorexic, undernourished child.
    B. a malnourished child with a swollen abdomen.
    C. an overweight but undernourished child.
    D. a well-nourished, healthy child.

14. The child who receives a bone marrow transplant will require:
    A. meticulous skin care.
    B. multiple peripheral sites for intravenous therapy.
    C. less chemotherapy prior to the transplant.
    D. a room with laminar air flow.

15. Currently the term *acute* is used in the classification of the leukemias to imply that:
    A. there is an increased number of abnormal mature cells present in the bone marrow.
    B. the course of the disease progresses slowly.
    C. the course of the disease involves rapid deterioration.
    D. there is an increased number of immature blast cells present in the bone marrow.

16. Which one of the following children with acute lymphoblastic leukemia has the BEST prognosis?
    A. a 1-year-old boy with a leukocyte count of $30,000/mm^3$
    B. a 6-year-old boy with a leukocyte count of $120,000/mm^3$
    C. a 1-year-old girl with a leukocyte count of $30,000/mm^3$
    D. a 6-year-old girl with a leukocyte count of $120,000/mm^3$

17. Staging the child by using initial white blood cell count, the patient's age and sex, and the histologic type of the disease is used to:
    A. determine potential chemotherapy side effects.
    B. estimate long-term survival.
    C. make a definitive diagnosis of leukemia.
    D. determine whether metastases have occurred.

18. To attempt to prevent central nervous system invasion of malignant cells, children with leukemia usually receive prophylactic:
    A. cranial/spinal irradiation.
    B. intravenous steroid therapy.
    C. intrathecal chemotherapy.
    D. intravenous methotrexate and cytarabine.

19. The fact that 95% of children with acute lymphoid leukemia will achieve an initial remission should be interpreted as:
    A. the percentage of children who will live five years or longer.
    B. an estimate that applies to children treated with the most successful protocols since diagnosis.
    C. the number to use only for the low-risk group of children.
    D. the estimate that may be used to determine the probability of a cure.

20. Hodgkin disease increases in incidence in children:
    A. under the age of 5 years.
    B. between the ages of 5 and 10 years.
    C. between the ages of 11 and 14 years.
    D. between the ages of 15 and 19 years.

21. Using present treatment protocols, prognosis for Hodgkin disease may be estimated with:
    A. the Ann Arbor Staging Classification.
    B. histologic staging.
    C. degree of tumor burden.
    D. initial leukocyte count.

22. A child with Hodgkin disease who has lesions in the left and the right supraclavicular areas, the mediastinum, and the lungs would be classified as:
    A. Stage I.
    B. Stage II.
    C. Stage III.
    D. Stage IV.

23. The Sternberg-Reed cell is a significant finding, because it:
    A. is absent in all diseases other than Hodgkin disease.
    B. is absent in all diseases other than the lymphomas.
    C. eliminates the need for laparotomy to determine the stage of the disease.
    D. is absent in all lymphomas other than Hodgkin disease.

24. The child who is scheduled for a lymphangiography examination should be told:
    A. to restrict his/her activity to quiet play after the test.
    B. the test will take about two hours.
    C. the test often takes four to five hours.
    D. to take nothing by mouth for at least eight hours before the test.

25. Match the major brain tumor of childhood with its characteristics.

A. medulloblastoma   _____ poor prognosis, because tumor is located in vital brain centers

B. cerebellar astrocytoma   _____ the most common pediatric brain tumor; infiltrates brain paren-chyma without distinct boundaries

C. low-grade astrocytoma

                              _____ usually invades the ventricles and obstructs the cerebrospinal fluid flow

D. ependymoma

E. brainstem glioma   _____ slow-growing tumor (if low-grade); has a 70% to 90% likelihood of cure (without residual tumor postoperatively)

                              _____ fast-growing, highly malignant tumor with a high risk of recurrence

26. The early signs and symptoms of brain tumor in the infant:
    A. are similar to those of a young child's.
    B. may be undetectable while the sutures are open.
    C. will be demonstrated as vomiting after feedings.
    D. will be demonstrated as headache and vomiting.

27. Which one of the following surgical techniques involves the use of computerized tomography and magnetic resonance imaging during the surgery?
    A. sclerotherapy
    B. microsurgery
    C. laser surgery
    D. stereotactic surgery

28. Which one of the following signs is MOST abnormal in the child who had surgery for a brain tumor 24 hours ago?
    A. The child is comatose.
    B. There is serous sanguinous drainage on the dressing.
    C. There is colorless drainage on the dressing.
    D. There is decreased muscle strength.

29. If a child vomits in the postoperative period following surgery for a brain tumor, it may predispose the child to:
    A. incisional rupture.
    B. increased intracranial pressure.
    C. aspiration.
    D. all of the above.

30. Neuroblastoma is often classified as a silent tumor because:
    A. diagnosis is not usually made until after metastasis.
    B. the primary site is intracranial.
    C. the primary site is the bone marrow.
    D. diagnosis is made based on the location of the primary site.

31. The most common bone cancer in children, osteogenic sarcoma, has a peak incidence at the age of:
    A. birth to 4 years.
    B. 4 years to 8 years.
    C. 8 years to 10 years.
    D. over 10 years.

32. Treatment for Ewing sarcoma would usually include:
    A. radiation alone.
    B. radiation and chemotherapy.
    C. amputation and chemotherapy.
    D. chemotherapy alone.

33. Wilm's tumor in children is treated with:
    A. chemotherapy and radiation.
    B. surgery and radiation.
    C. surgery and chemotherapy.
    D. surgery alone.

34. Rhabdomyosarcoma is a:
    A. malignant bone neoplasm.
    B. nonmalignant soft tissue tumor.
    C. nonmalignant solid tumor.
    D. malignant solid tumor of the soft tissue.

35. Bilateral malignant retinoblastoma is almost always considered to be transmitted by:
    A. an autosomal dominant trait.
    B. a somatic mutation.
    C. a chromosomal aberration.
    D. an autosomal recessive trait.

36. Instructions for the parents of a child who has an eye enucleation performed should be based on the fact that:
    A. there will be a cavity in the skull where the eye was.
    B. the child's face may be edematous and ecchymotic.
    C. the eyelids will be open and the surgical site will be sunken.
    D. all of the above

37. A nodule discovered on an adolescent male's testicle should be evaluated, because a tumor in this location:
    A. usually causes infertility.
    B. in this age group is usually malignant.
    C. has usually metastasized by the time of discovery.
    D. could not be felt using testicular self-examination.

❖ Critical Thinking ❖
Case Study

Cory Henderson is a 6-year-old child who is diagnosed with acute lymphoid leukemia. She receives chemotherapy regularly. Her parents are divorced and she is an only child. She lives with her mother and rarely sees her father.

Cory attends first grade when she can. She had little difficulty with school before her diagnosis, but lately she has had trouble keeping up with the activities because she is so tired.

38. Today Cory arrives at the chemotherapy clinic for her regular medication regimen. A complete blood count shows that her white blood count is lower than expected. The BEST nursing diagnosis for the nurse to use for Cory today based on the above information would be:
    A. altered family processes related to the therapy.
    B. high risk for hemorrhagic cystitis related to white cell proliferation.
    C. high risk for infection related to depressed body defenses.
    D. altered mucous membranes related to administration of chemotherapy.

39. Cory's mother tells the nurse she has noticed that after the chemotherapy, Cory's appetite is usually quite poor. She knows that nutrition is essential, so she is trying everything to get Cory to eat even during those times when she is nauseated after the chemotherapy. Strategies the nurse might suggest would include:
A. have Cory gargle with viscous Xylocaine to relieve pain.
B. permit only nutritious snacks.
C. establish regular meal times.
D. offer small snacks frequently.

40. To plan for the body image disturbance related to loss of hair, moon face, and debilitation, which of the following actions by Cory's mother would be considered beneficial?
A. Emphasize the benefits of the therapy.
B. Encourage Cory to select a wig to wear.
C. Suggest that Cory keep her hair long for as long as possible.
D. all of the above

41. Which one of the following expected outcomes would be appropriate for the nurse to measure Cory's mother's progress toward coping with the possibility of her child's death?
A. Cory's mother is able to talk to the staff about her fear of living without her daughter.
B. Cory's mother is able to verbalize an understanding of the procedures and tests that have been performed.
C. Cory's mother is able to provide the care at home that is needed.
D. Cory's mother complies with the suggestions the nurses make.

❖ Crossword Puzzle ❖

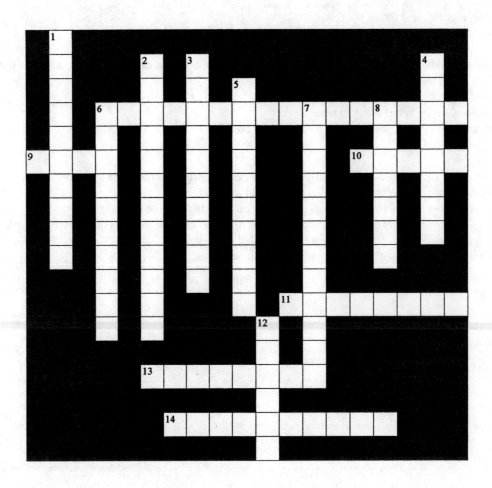

Across

6. Reduction in the blood-forming cells made in the bone marrow
9. Acute nonlymphocytic leukemia
10. Common acute lymphoblastic leukemic antigen
11. Written statement of a specific treatment plan
13. The study of cancer
14. A second lesion developing away from the primary lesion

Down

1. A substance that causes cancer
2. Treatment with chemical substances having a specific effect on a disease
3. Treatment that uses BRM to combat malignancy
4. A mass of newly formed tissue
5. Rapid breakdown of malignant cells (2 words)
6. A cancerous condition
7. Treatment by means of irradiation
8. Defining the phase of a disease
12. Removal of tissue for examination

❖ CHAPTER 37
The Child with Cerebral Dysfunction

1. Cerebral blood flow, oxygen consumption, and brain growth are all:
   A. less in adults than in children.
   B. greater in adults than in children.
   C. greater in adults than in infants.
   D. less in infants than in children.

2. Match the structure of the brain with its function.

   A. parietal lobes

   B. temporal lobes

   C. cerebrum

   D. basal ganglia

   E. thalamus

   F. brainstem

   G. mesencephalon (midbrain)

   H. medulla

   I. cerebellum

   J. frontal lobes

   K. occipital lobe

   L. diencephalon

   M. hypothalamus

   N. pons

   _____ receive/interpret stimuli for all of the senses

   _____ contains the vasomotor cranial nerves

   _____ contains pneumotaxic center and controls respiration

   _____ necessary for coordination and balance

   _____ vital control center of involuntary functions (temperature regulation)

   _____ All cranial nerves except cranial nerve I arise from this structure.

   _____ center for consciousness, thought, memory, sensory input, and motor activity

   _____ receives stimuli for vision and spatial orientation

   _____ connects the forebrain to the hindbrain

   _____ a major relay station for sensory impulses to the cerebral cortex

   _____ controls motor activity, social interaction, and abstract thinking

   _____ causes inhibition of muscle tone throughout the body

   _____ contains fibers that compose the reticular activating system

   _____ important for interpretation of sensation

3. The blood-brain barrier in an infant is:
   A. less permeable than in the adult.
   B. impermeable to protein.
   C. impermeable to glucose.
   D. permeable to large molecules.

4. Which one of the following signs is used to evaluate increased intracranial pressure in the infant but not in the older child?
   A. projectile vomiting
   B. headache
   C. nonpulsating fontanel
   D. pulsating fontanel

5. Which of the following indicators is BEST to use to determine the depth of the comatose state?
   A. motor activity
   B. level of consciousness
   C. reflexes
   D. vital signs

6. The guidelines for establishing brain death in children:
   A. differ from age to age.
   B. are the same as in the adult.
   C. all require an observation period of at least seven days.
   D. all require an observation period of at least 48 hours.

7. After a seizure in a child over 3 years of age, the Babinski reflex often:
   A. remains positive.
   B. changes from positive to negative.
   C. changes from negative to positive.
   D. remains negative.

8. Which one of the following reflex patterns would be considered MOST healthy in young infants?
   A. negative Moro reflex and a positive tonic neck reflex
   B. negative Moro reflex and a negative tonic neck reflex
   C. positive Moro reflex and a positive tonic neck reflex
   D. positive Moro reflex and a negative tonic neck reflex

9. Which one of the following tests should NOT be used if the patient has an increase in intracranial pressure?
   A. lumbar puncture
   B. subdural tap
   C. computed tomography
   D. digital subtraction angiography

10. Which one of the following nursing observations would usually indicate pain in a comatose child?
    A. increased flaccidity
    B. increased oxygen saturation
    C. decreased blood pressure
    D. increased agitation

11. Intracranial pressure monitoring has been found to be useful in pediatric critical care to:
    A. determine the outcome of a pediatric neurologic injury.
    B. evaluate children with Glasgow Coma Scales under seven.
    C. give an indication of the severity of the neurologic insult in the initial evaluation of a child.
    D. all of the above

12. Which one of the following activities has been shown to increase intracranial pressure?
    A. using earplugs to eliminate noise
    B. range-of-motion exercises
    C. suctioning
    D. osmotherapy

13. If a child is permanently unconscious, it would be INAPPROPRIATE for the nurse to:
    A. permit the parents to bring a child's favorite toy.
    B. provide guidance and clarify information that the physician has already given.
    C. suggest the parents plan for periodic relief from the continual care of their child.
    D. use reflexive muscle contractions as a sign of hope for recovery.

14. Which of the following neurological conditions occurs more often in children with a head injury than in adults with a head injury?
    A. cerebral hyperemia
    B. hypoxic brain damage
    C. cerebral edema
    D. subdural hemorrhage

15. Epidural hemorrhage is less common in children under 2 years of age than in adults because:
    A. the middle meningeal artery is embedded in the bone surface of the skull until approximately 2 years of age.
    B. fractures are less likely to lacerate the middle meningeal artery in children under 2 years of age.
    C. separation of the dura from bleeding is more likely to occur in children than in adults.
    D. there is an increased tendency for the skull to fracture in children under 2 years of age.

16. The goal in the management of a child with a head injury is to:
    A. eliminate ischemic brain damage.
    B. eliminate original primary insult.
    C. care for the secondary brain injuries.
    D. all of the above

17. Which one of the following interventions would NOT be considered part of the emergency treatment of a child with a head injury?
    A. Administer analgesics.
    B. Check pupil reaction to light.
    C. Stabilize the neck and spine.
    D. Check level of consciousness.

18. After craniocerebral trauma, children usually have a:
    A. lower incidence of psychological disturbances than adults.
    B. higher mortality rate than adults.
    C. less favorable prognosis than adults.
    D. higher incidence of psychological disturbances than adults.

19. Family support for the child who has suffered head injury includes all of the following EXCEPT to encourage the parents to:
    A. hold and cuddle the child.
    B. bring familiar belongings into the child's room.
    C. make a tape recording of familiar voices/sounds.
    D. search for clues that the child is recovering.

20. Which of the following predictors was NOT associated with prognosis for a near-drowning victim in the study conducted by Quan and Kinder in 1992?
    A. the cardiac rhythm
    B. the degree of acidosis upon admission
    C. the response of the pupils to light
    D. the length of time the child was submerged

21. The etiology of bacterial meningitis has changed in recent years due to the:
    A. increased surveillance of tuberculosis.
    B. increased awareness of rubella vaccines.
    C. routine use of *H. influenzae* type B vaccine.
    D. routine use of hepatitis B vaccine.

22. The MOST common mode of transmission for bacterial meningitis is:
    A. vascular dissemination of a respiratory tract infection.
    B. direct implantation from an invasive procedure.
    C. direct extension from an infection in the mastoid sinuses.
    D. direct extension from an infection in the nasal sinuses.

23. Secondary problems from bacterial meningitis are MOST likely to occur in the:
    A. child with meningococcal meningitis.
    B. infant under 2 months of age.
    C. infant over 2 months of age.
    D. child with *H. influenzae* type B meningitis.

24. Which one of the following types of meningitis is self-limiting and least serious?
    A. meningococcal meningitis
    B. tuberculous meningitis
    C. *H. influenzae* meningitis
    D. nonbacterial (aseptic) meningitis

25. Which one of the following types of encephalitis occurs in children one-third of the time?
    A. herpes simplex
    B. measles
    C. mumps
    D. rubella

26. Which of the following domestic animals should be the target of a community rabies vaccination program?
    A. dogs
    B. hamsters
    C. cats
    D. parakeets

27. For the control of rabies, The World Health Organization recommends:
    A. mass immunization using human rabies immune globulin.
    B. administration of human diploid cell rabies vaccine according to schedule for three months after the exposure.
    C. mass immunization using human diploid cell rabies vaccine.
    D. administration of human rabies immune globulin 90 days after the exposure.

28. The link between aspirin and Reye's Syndrome:
    A. is firmly established.
    B. is a cause-and-effect relationship.
    C. has alerted the public to the hazard of drugs.
    D. all of the above

29. Symptoms that are similar to those of Reye's syndrome have occurred during viral illnesses when the child was given an:
    A. antiemetic drug.
    B. analgesic drug.
    C. antiepileptic drug.
    D. antiarrhythmic drug.

30. Most children with epilepsy have:
    A. focal seizures.
    B. generalized seizures.
    C. partial seizures.
    D. partial seizures that become generalized.

31. One action the nurse may take to provide a clue to the origin of a seizure is to:
    A. attempt to place an airway in the mouth.
    B. gently open the eyes to observe their movement.
    C. administer antiepileptic and observe the effect.
    D. all of the above

32. Which one of the following types of seizures is MOST common in children between the ages of 4 and 12 years?
    A. generalized seizures
    B. absence seizures
    C. atonic seizures
    D. jackknife seizures

33. Which one of the following antiepileptic drugs acts only on a developing brain and therefore is used for infantile spasms?
    A. adrenocorticotropic hormone
    B. valproic acid
    C. ethosuximide
    D. felbamate

34. Therapy for epilepsy should include:
    A. short-term drug therapy.
    B. combination drug therapy.
    C. only one drug, if possible.
    D. drugs that correct the brain wave pattern.

35. A poor prognosis for the child with status epilepticus is associated with:
    A. previous developmental delays.
    B. previous neurologic abnormalities.
    C. concurrent serious illness.
    D. all of the above.

36. Nursing intervention for a child during a tonic-clonic seizure should include attempts to:
    A. halt the seizure as soon as it begins.
    B. restrain the child.
    C. remain calm and observe the child.
    D. place an oral airway in the child's mouth.

37. To prevent submersion injuries in children with epilepsy, the child should be instructed to:
    A. never go swimming.
    B. take showers.
    C. wear a bicycle helmet.
    D. all of the above

38. In most children who have a febrile seizure, the temperature factor that triggers the seizure tends to be the:
    A. rapidity of the temperature elevation.
    B. duration of the temperature elevation.
    C. height of the temperature elevation.
    D. any of the above

39. When a child has a febrile seizure, it is important for the parents to know that the child will:
    A. probably not develop epilepsy.
    B. most likely develop epilepsy.
    C. most likely develop neurologic damage.
    D. usually need tepid sponge baths to control fever.

40. In most cases, chronic recurrent headaches of childhood represent:
    A. tension.
    B. seizures.
    C. intracranial disease.
    D. migraine.

41. Treatment for migraine headaches in children usually includes:
    A. ergots.
    B. opioids.
    C. acetaminophen.
    D. all of the above.

❖ Critical Thinking ❖
Case Study

Jackson Smith was riding his bike in the street by his house when he was hit by a car. He is 9 years old. He was not wearing a helmet at the time. He has been unconscious since the accident eight hours ago. His mother and father both work full-time, and there are five other siblings at home ranging in age from 7 to 19 years old.

42. Based on the above information, which of the following nursing diagnoses would have the highest priority?
    A. high risk for impaired skin integrity related to immobility
    B. self-care deficit related to inability to feed himself
    C. altered family processes related to a permanent disability
    D. high risk for aspiration related to impaired motor function

43. In order to effectively deal with the altered family processes related to the hospitalization, the nurse should:
    A. provide information about bicycle safety helmets.
    B. encourage expression of feelings.
    C. encourage the family to provide Jackson's hygiene needs.
    D. provide auditory stimulation for Jackson.

44. In order to help Jackson receive appropriate sensory stimulation, the nurse should:
    A. hang a black and white mobile above his bed.
    B. hang a calendar at the foot of his bed.
    C. encourage the family to bring a tape of his favorite music.
    D. administer pain medications as needed.

45. Jackson's parents visit him every day, but never together. The nurse should be concerned about:
    A. marital problems that usually occur during stressful times like this.
    B. whether Jackson's parents are able to receive adequate support for each other with this arrangement.
    C. whether Jackson's siblings are being adequately cared for.
    D. all of the above.

❖ Crossword Puzzle ❖

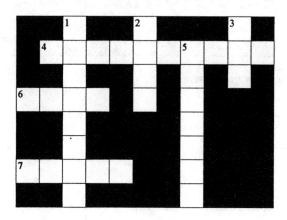

Across

4. Involuntary muscle contraction and relaxation
6. Adrenocorticotropic hormone
7. Syndrome of inappropriate antidiuretic hormone

Down

1. Period following a seizure
2. A sensation that may precede an attack of migraine or an epileptic seizure
3. Level of consciousness
5. A sudden attack

❖ CHAPTER 38
The Child with Endocrine Dysfunction

1. List the three components of the endocrine system.

   _____

   _____

   _____

2. A hormone that produces its effect on a specific tissue would be classified as a _____ hormone.

3. Identify the target tissue or gland for each of the following hormones; then match the hormone with its effect.

Hormone	Target Tissue or Gland	Hormone's Effect
A. thyroid-stimulating hormone	A. _____	_____ increases reabsorption of water
B. luteinizing hormone	B. _____	_____ promotes growth of bone and soft tissue
C. somatotropic hormone	C. _____	_____ stimulates the secretion of glucocorticoids
D. gonadotropin	D. _____	_____ initiates spermatogenesis
E. melanocyte-stimulating hormone	E. _____	_____ regulates metabolic rate
F. adrenocorticotropic hormone	F. _____	_____ maintains corpus luteum during pregnancy
G. antidiuretic hormone	G. _____	_____ promotes pigmentation of the skin
H. follicle-stimulating hormone	H. _____	_____ causes the let-down reflex
I. oxytocin	I. _____	_____ produces sex hormones
J. prolactin	J. _____	_____ stimulates the secretion of testosterone in the male

4. Match the hormone or gland with its effect.

A. parathyroid _____ prepares uterus for fertilized ovum

B. cortisol _____ influences development of secondary sex characteristics

C. aldosterone _____ promotes breast development during puberty

D. thyroid _____ inhibits the secretion of insulin and glycogen

E. androgen _____ promotes normal fat protein and carbohydrate metabolism

F. glucagon _____ produces vasoconstriction and raises blood pressure

G. epinephrine _____ stimulates renal tubules to reabsorb sodium

H. progesterone _____ stimulates testes to produce spermatozoa

I. insulin _____ regulates metabolic rate

J. estrogen _____ promotes glucose transport into the cells

K. testosterone _____ promotes reabsorption of sodium and excretion of phosphorous

5. The difference between panhypopituitarism and idiopathic hypopituitarism is that:
A. idiopathic hypopituitarism is caused by a tumor.
B. the incidence of idiopathic hypopituitarism is higher in girls.
C. panhypopituitarism usually has a cause that is known.
D. panhypopituitarism is the cause of short stature in most children whose height is in the lower percentiles.

6. A child with growth hormone deficiency will exhibit the signs of:
A. retarded height and weight.
B. abnormal skeletal proportions.
C. malnutrition.
D. retarded height, but not necessarily retarded weight.

7. In a child with hypopituitarism, the growth hormone levels would usually be:
A. elevated after 20 minutes of strenuous exercise.
B. elevated 45 to 90 minutes after the onset of sleep.
C. lower in an overnight urine specimen.
D. rapidly increased in response to insulin.

8. The appropriate treatment of choice for the child with idiopathic hypopituitarism may be:
A. biosynthetic growth hormone.
B. human growth hormone.
C. surgical removal of the tumor.
D. any of the above.

9. Which one of the following statements about growth hormone replacement therapy in the child with idiopathic hypo-pituitarism is TRUE?
A. Therapy will continue for life.
B. Therapy will not result in achievement of a normal familial height.
C. Therapy requires subcutaneous injection.
D. Therapy requires intramuscular injection.

10. Provocative testing for diagnosis of hypopituitarism may require that the nurse monitor the child's:
    A. calcium levels.
    B. phosphorous levels.
    C. glucose levels.
    D. hemoglobin levels.

11. Explain the difference between acromegaly and the pituitary hyperfunction that would not be considered acromegaly.

    _____

    _____

    _____

12. Parents of the child with precocious puberty need to know that:
    A. dress and activities should be aligned with the child's sexual development.
    B. heterosexual interest will usually be advanced.
    C. the child's mental age is congruent with the chronological age.
    D. overt manifestations of affection represent sexual advances.

13. Desmopressin acetate, used to treat diabetes insipidus, may be administered:
    A. by mouth.
    B. intranasally.
    C. topically.
    D. all of the above

14. The MOST common cause of thyroid disease in children and adolescents is:
    A. Hashimoto's disease.
    B. Grave's disease.
    C. goiter.
    D. thyrotoxicosis.

15. The initial treatment for the child with hyperthyroidism would MOST likely be:
    A. subtotal thyroidectomy.
    B. total thyroidectomy.
    C. ablation with radioactive iodide.
    D. administration of thyroid hormone.

16. When a thyroidectomy is planned, the nurse should explain to the child that:
    A. iodine preparations will be mixed with flavored foods and then eaten.
    B. he/she will need to hyperextend his/her neck postoperatively.
    C. the skin, not the throat, will be cut.
    D. laryngospasm can be a life-threatening complication.

17. The child with hypoparathyroidism will usually exhibit:
    A. short, stubby fingers.
    B. dimpling of the skin over the knuckles.
    C. thin, brittle nails.
    D. a short, thick neck.

18. A common cause of secondary hyperparathyroidism is:
    A. maternal hyperparathyroidism.
    B. chronic renal disease.
    C. an adenoma.
    D. renal rickets.

19. Hypofunction of the adrenal medulla results in:
    A. release of epinephrine and norepinephrine from the sympathetic nervous system.
    B. pheochromocytoma.
    C. adrenal crisis.
    D. myxedema.

20. Diagnosis of acute adrenocortical insufficiency is made based on:
    A. elevated plasma cortisol levels.
    B. the history and physical examination.
    C. depressed plasma cortisol levels.
    D. depressed aldosterone levels.

21. The parents of a child who has Addison's disease should be instructed to:
    A. use extra hydrocortisone only for crises.
    B. discontinue the child's cortisone if side effects develop.
    C. decrease the cortisone dose during times of stress.
    D. report signs of Cushing's syndrome to the physician.

22. Which one of the following tests is particularly useful in diagnosing congenital adrenogenital hyperplasia?
    A. chromosome typing
    B. pelvic ultrasound
    C. pelvic x-ray
    D. testosterone levels

23. The temporary treatment for hyperaldosteronism prior to surgery would usually involve administration of:
    A. spironolactone.
    B. phentolamine.
    C. furosemide.
    D. phenoxybenzamine.

24. Definitive treatment for pheochromocytoma consists of:
    A. surgical removal of the thyroid.
    B. administration of potassium.
    C. surgical removal of the tumor.
    D. administration of beta blockers.

25. Most children with diabetes mellitus tend to exhibit characteristics of:
    A. maturity-onset diabetes of youth.
    B. gestational diabetes.
    C. type II diabetes.
    D. type I diabetes.

26. The currently accepted etiology of insulin-dependent diabetes takes into account:
    A. genetic factors.
    B. autoimmune mechanisms.
    C. environmental factors.
    D. all of the above.

27. An early sign of insulin-dependent diabetes in the adolescent would be:
    A. a vaginal candida infection.
    B. obesity.
    C. Kussmaul's respirations.
    D. all of the above.

28. Glycosylated hemoglobin is an acceptable method to use to:
    A. diagnose diabetes mellitus.
    B. assess the control of diabetes.
    C. assess oxygen saturation of the hemoglobin.
    D. determine blood glucose levels most accurately.

29. The MOST common acute complication of diabetes that a young child encounters is:
    A. retinopathy.
    B. ketoacidosis.
    C. hypoglycemia.
    D. hyperosmolar non-ketotic coma.

30. Principles of managing diabetes during illness include all of the following EXCEPT:
    A. monitor blood glucose every four hours.
    B. use a sliding scale of regular insulin.
    C. omit insulin when excessive vomiting occurs.
    D. use simple sugars as carbohydrate exchanges.

31. Diabetic ketoacidosis in children with diabetes mellitus is:
    A. the most common chronic complication.
    B. usually precipitated by a variety of factors.
    C. a life-threatening complication.
    D. all of the above.

32. In regard to meal planning for the child with diabetes mellitus:
    A. fast foods must be eliminated.
    B. foods must always be weighed and measured.
    C. the exchange list is limited to one type of food.
    D. foods with sorbitol are not recommended.

33. In regard to insulin administration:
    A. insulin should never be premixed.
    B. insulin syringes should never be reused.
    C. insulin doses under 2 units should be diluted.
    D. an air bubble in the syringe is insignificant.

34. Exercise for the child with diabetes mellitus is:
    A. restricted to noncontact sports.
    B. may require a decreased intake of food.
    C. may necessitate an increased insulin dose.
    D. may require an increased intake of food.

35. Problems of adjustment to diabetes are MOST likely to occur when diabetes is diagnosed in:
    A. infancy.
    B. adolescence.
    C. the toddler years.
    D. the school-age years.

❖ *Critical Thinking* ❖
Case Study

Rebecca Bennett is an 8-year-old who has just been diagnosed with diabetes mellitus. She is hospitalized with diabetic ketoacidosis and is beginning to learn about the disease process. Her parents are with her continuously. She has an identical twin sister who is staying with the maternal grandparents.

36. Mrs. Bennett is concerned that Rebecca's sister will also develop diabetes. Based on the above information, an acceptable response for the nurse to make would be to:
    A. reassure the parents that the disease is not contagious.
    B. discuss the hereditary and viral factors of type I diabetes.
    C. discuss the hereditary factors of type I diabetes.
    D. discuss the viral factors of type I diabetes.

37. Which one of the following nursing diagnoses is MOST likely to become a priority after the first few days of Rebecca's hospitalization?
    A. fluid volume deficit related to uncontrolled diabetes
    B. fluid volume excess related to hormonal disturbances
    C. impaired home maintenance management related to lack of knowledge
    D. impaired respiratory function related to fluid imbalance

38. In preparing the Bennett family for discharge, the nurse should plan to teach:
    A. only Rebecca how to inject insulin.
    B. only Rebecca's parents how to inject insulin.
    C. both Rebecca and her parents how to inject insulin.
    D. the family how to administer oral hypoglycemics.

39. To evaluate Rebecca's progress in relation to her diabetes management, the BEST measure would be Rebecca's:
    A. parents' verbalizations about the disease process.
    B. blood glucose levels.
    C. glycosylated hemoglobin values.
    D. demonstration of her insulin injection technique.

❖ Crossword Puzzle ❖

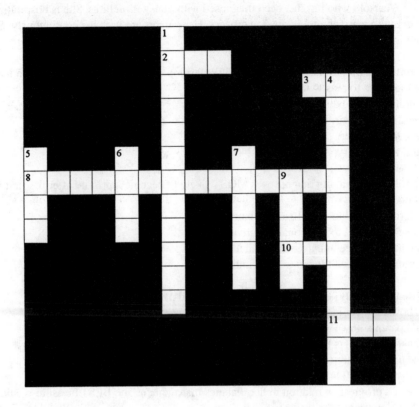

Across

2. Human lymphocyte antigen
3. Parathyroid hormone
8. Breakdown of glycogen to glucose
10. Diabetic ketoacidosis
11. Islet cell antibodies

Down

1. Facial muscle spasm (2 words)
4. Carpal spasm (2 words)
5. Home glucose blood monitoring
6. Maturity-onset diabetes of youth
7. The different forms of a gene
9. Syndrome of inappropriate ADH

❖ CHAPTER 39
The Child with Musculoskeletal or Articular Dysfunction

1. The neighbor of Jimmy, age 5, discovers him lying in the street next to his bicycle. The neighbor, who is a nurse, sends another witness to activate the Emergency Medical System while the nurse begins a primary assessment of Jimmy. Which one of the following BEST describes the primary assessment and its correct sequence?
   A. body inspection, head-to-toe survey, and airway patency
   B. airway patency, respiratory effectiveness, and circulatory status
   C. open airway, head-to-toe assessment for injuries, and chest compressions
   D. weight estimation, symptom analysis, and blood pressure measurement

2. Major consequences of immobilization in the pediatric patient include which one of the following?
   A. bone demineralization leading to osteoporosis
   B. orthostatic hypertension
   C. dependent edema in the lower extremities
   D. decrease in the metabolic rate

3. Nursing interventions aimed at preventing problems associated with immobilization include which one of the following?
   A. encouragement in self-care and allowing patients to do as much for themselves as they are able to perform
   B. fluid restrictions with strict intake and output
   C. limitation of active range-of-motion exercises to once per day
   D. decreased sensory stimulation to allow adequate rest

4. The fabrication and fitting of braces is termed _____. The fabrication and fitting of artificial limbs

   is termed _____.

5. Which one of the following is a complication of immobility that is easily prevented by an appropriate nursing intervention?
   A. disuse atrophy and loss of muscle mass
   B. constipation
   C. hypocalcemia
   D. pain

6. Which one of the following is NOT included in the teaching plan of a child with a brace or prosthesis?
   A. frequent assessment of all areas in contact with the brace for signs of skin irritation
   B. assessment of the stump area before application of the prosthesis
   C. Removal of the prosthesis is limited to bedtime unless skin breakage occurs.
   D. Protective clothing is used under the brace.

7. Bone healing is characteristically more rapid in children because:
   A. children have less constant muscle contraction associated with the fracture.
   B. children's fractures are less severe than adult's.
   C. children have an active growth plate that helps speed repair with deformity less likely to occur.
   D. children have thickened periosteum and more generous blood supply.

8. The method of fracture reduction is NOT determined by which one of the following?
   A. age of the child
   B. how the fracture occurred
   C. the degree of displacement
   D. the amount of edema

9. Match the term with its description.

   A. diaphysis   _____ fracture with an open wound from which the bone has protruded

   B. epiphysis   _____ major portion of the long bone

   C. epiphyseal plate   _____ fracture fragments are separated

   D. complete   _____ fracture fragments remain attached

   E. incomplete   _____ located at the ends of the long bones

   F. transverse   _____ also called the growth plate because it plays a major role in the longitudinal
                                    growth of the developing child
   G. simple
                           _____ fracture that is crosswise, at right angles to the long axis of the bone
   H. open
                           _____ small fragments of bone are broken from the fractured shaft and lie in sur-
   I. complicated   rounding tissue

   J. comminuted   _____ bone fragments cause damage to surrounding organs or tissue

   K. greenstick   _____ fracture has not produced a break in the skin

   L. buckle   _____ appears as a raising or bulging at the site of the fracture

   M. bends   _____ occurs more commonly in the ulna and fibula and can produce some de-
                                    formity

                           _____ occurs when a bone is angulated beyond the limits of bending

10. Emergency treatment for the child with a fracture does NOT include:
    A. assessing for pain, point tenderness, pulse distal to the fracture site, pallor, paresthesia, and paralysis.
    B. immobilization of the limb.
    C. pushing the protruding bone under the skin.
    D. applying cold to the injured area.

11. An appropriate nursing intervention for the care of a child with an extremity in a new cast is:
    A. keeping the cast covered with a sheet.
    B. using the fingertips when handling the cast to prevent pressure areas.
    C. using heated fans or dryers to circulate air and speed the cast-drying process.
    D. turning the child at least every two hours to help dry the cast evenly.

12. To reduce anxiety in the child undergoing cast removal, which one of the following nursing interventions would the
    nurse expect to be LEAST effective?
    A. Demonstrate how the cast cutter works to the child before beginning the procedure.
    B. Use the analogy of having fingernails or hair cut.
    C. Explain that it will take only a few minutes.
    D. Give continual reassurance that all is going well and that the child's behavior is accepted during the removal pro-
       cess.

13. The nurse is caring for 7-year-old Charles after insertion of skeletal traction. Which one of the following is CONTRA-INDICATED?
    A. Gently massage over pressure areas to stimulate circulation.
    B. Release the traction when repositioning Charles in bed.
    C. Inspect pin sites for bleeding or infection.
    D. Assess for alterations in neurovascular status.

14. Match the type of traction with its description.

    A. Dunlop traction   _____ insertion of a wire or pin into the bone

    B. Bryant traction   _____ used to realign bone fragments for cast application

    C. Buck extension   _____ applied when there is minimum displacement and little muscle
                                                    spasticity, but contraindicated when there is associated skin damage
    D. Russell traction
                                            _____ treatment of fractures of the humerus when the arm is suspended
    E. 90-degree—90-degree traction   horizontally

    F. balance suspension traction   _____ a type of running traction where the pull is in only one direction

    G. Thomas splint   _____ uses skin traction on the lower leg and a padded sling under the knee

    H. Pearson attachment   _____ a type of skin traction with the leg in an extended position; used
                                                    primarily for short-term immobilization
    I. cervical traction
                                            _____ skeletal traction where the lower leg is put in a boot cast or sup-
    J. manual traction   ported in a sling and a pin is placed in the distal fragment of the
                                                    femur
    K. skin traction
                                            _____ used with or without skin or skeletal traction; suspends the leg in a
    L. skeletal traction   flexed position to relax the hip and hamstring muscles

                                            _____ extends from the groin to midair above the foot

                                            _____ supports the lower leg

                                            _____ accomplished by insertion of Crutchfield tongs through burr holes

15. The nurse is assessing Carol, age 8, for complications related to her recent fracture and the application of a flexion cast to her forearm and elbow. Carol is crying with pain, the nurse is unable to locate pulses in the affected extremity, and there is lack of sensitivity to the area as well as some edema. Which one of the following would the nurse suspect as MOST likely to be occurring?
    A. This is a normal occurrence for the first few hours following application of traction.
    B. Volkmann contracture
    C. nerve compression syndrome
    D. epiphyseal damage

16. Nursing interventions for the child following surgical amputation of a lower extremity include:
    A. applying special elastic bandaging to the stump using a circular pattern to decrease stump edema.
    B. keeping the stump elevated for at least 72 hours post surgery.
    C. encouraging the child to lie prone at least three times a day, increasing the time prone to tolerance of an hour at a time.
    D. recognizing that the child is only trying to gain the nurse's attention when the child says there is pain in the missing limb.

17. Immediate treatment of sprains and strains includes:
    A. rest and cold application.
    B. disregarding the pain and "working out" the sprain or strain.
    C. rest, elevation, and pain medication.
    D. compression of the area and heat application.

18. Major sprains or tears to the ligamentous tissue rarely occur in growing children because the _____

    are stronger than bone. The _____ and the _____ _____ are
    the weakest part of the bone and the usual site of injury.

19. Identify the following statements as either TRUE or FALSE.

    _____ Achilles tendonitis is caused by repeated forcible traction on the short tendon.

    _____ Jumper's knee is caused by epiphysitis of the calcaneus.

    _____ Osgood-Schlatter disease may present with pain and tenderness over the tibial tubercle and an over-
    prominence of involved tubercle.

    _____ Little League elbow presents with pain in the elbow, aggravated by use, and is caused from repetitive
    strain on lateral epicondylitis.

    _____ Children are less vulnerable to heat injury than adults because of their greater ratio of surface area to
    body mass and reduced production of metabolic heat for body mass.

    _____ Heat cramps are caused by calcium depletion during vigorous exercise in a hot environment.

    _____ Heat exhaustion occurs from excessive loss of fluids during exercise in a hot environment. Symptoms
    include thirst, headache, fatigue, dizziness, anxiety, and nausea or vomiting.

    _____ The child with heat exhaustion should have external cooling applied with cold towels immediately.

    _____ Heatstroke represents a failure of normal thermoregulatory mechanisms. Onset is rapid and disorienta-
    tion is present, along with a temperature in excess of 104° F.

    _____ Salt tablets are rarely needed and may actually do harm by increasing dehydration.

    _____ Any athlete who loses more than 3% of body weight in an exercise session should not return to activity
    until the fluid is restored.

    _____ It is not necessary to counsel female athletes about pregnancy prevention because they have delayed
    menarche.

    _____ Drug misuse by athletes most often includes psychomotor stimulants and anabolic steroids.

20. The condition recognized in the infant with limited neck motion, where the neck is flexed and turned to the affected
    side as a result of shortening of the sternocleidomastoid muscle, is:
    A. torticollis.
    B. paralysis of the brachial nerve.
    C. Legg-Calvé-Perthes disease.
    D. a self-limiting injury.

21. Ben, age 7, is diagnosed with Legg-Calvé-Perthes disease. Which one of the following manifestations is NOT consistent with this diagnosis?
   A. intermittent appearance of a limp on the affected side
   B. hip soreness, ache, or stiffness that can be constant or intermittent
   C. pain and limp most evident on arising and at the end of a long day of activities
   D. specific history of injury to the area

22. Slipped femoral capital epiphysis is suspected when:
   A. an adolescent or preadolescent begins to limp and complains of pain in the hip continuously or intermittently.
   B. examination reveals no restriction on internal rotation or adduction but restriction on external rotation.
   C. referred pain goes into the sacral and lumbar areas.
   D. all of the above

23. An accentuation of the lumbar curvature beyond physiologic limits is termed _____. An abnormally increased convex angulation in the curvature of the thoracic spine is termed _____.

   _____ is the forward slipping of one vertebral body on another, usually L5 and S1.

24. Diagnostic evaluation is important for early recognition of scoliosis. Which one of the following is the CORRECT procedure for the school nurse conducting this examination?
   A. View the child standing and walking fully clothed to look for uneven hanging of clothing.
   B. View all children from the left and right side to look mainly for asymmetry of the hip height.
   C. Completely undress all children before the examination.
   D. View the child who is wearing underpants from behind and when the child bends forward.

25. Marilyn, age 13, has been diagnosed with scoliosis and placed in a Milwaukee brace. Marilyn asks the nurse about the brace and how long she has to wear it. What is the BEST response?
   A. "The brace will need to be worn only until you have corrective surgery."
   B. "The brace will need to be worn approximately 23 hours a day to halt or slow the progression of the curvature."
   C. "The brace will not need to be worn to school, only at home, and you will need to sleep in the brace."
   D. "You will need to get specific information about your schedule from your doctor."

26. Nursing implementation directed toward nonsurgical management in a teenager with scoliosis primarily includes:
   A. promoting self-esteem and positive body image.
   B. preventing immobility.
   C. promoting adequate nutrition.
   D. preventing infection.

27. The plan of care for the child during the acute phase of osteomyelitis always includes:
   A. performing wound irrigations.
   B. maintaining IV infusion site.
   C. isolation of the child.
   D. passive range-of-motion exercises for the affected area.

28. Nursing considerations for the patient diagnosed with osteogenesis imperfecta include:
   A. preventing fractures by careful handling.
   B. providing nonjudgmental support while parents are dealing with accusations of child abuse.
   C. providing guidelines to the parents in planning suitable activities that promote optimum development.
   D. all of the above.

29. Which of the following nursing goals is MOST appropriate for the child with juvenile rheumatoid arthritis?
   A. Child will exhibit signs of reduced joint inflammation and adequate joint function.
   B. Child will exhibit no signs of impaired skin integrity due to rash.
   C. Child will exhibit normal weight and nutritional status.
   D. Child will exhibit no alteration in respiratory patterns or respiratory infection.

30. The majority of children with clinical manifestations of systemic lupus erythematosus present with which one of the following?
   A. Raynaud phenomenon, especially of the feet and legs
   B. development of herpes simplex in dry, cracked skin areas
   C. cutaneous involvement including skin disease as the chief complaint
   D. patchy areas of alopecia without remission

❖ Critical Thinking ❖
Case Study

Sandy, age 8, has developed joint and leg pain, some joint swelling, fever, malaise, and pleuritis. The physician has ordered laboratory testing to include sedimentation rate, rheumatoid factor, and a complete blood count. Tentative diagnosis has been established as juvenile arthritis, systemic onset.

31. If the diagnosis is correct, which of the following would represent the expected laboratory results?
   A. leukocytosis
   B. elevated sedimentation rate
   C. negative rheumatoid factor
   D. all of the above

32. The primary group of drugs prescribed for juvenile arthritis is nonsteroidal antiinflammatory drugs. Education regarding the use of these drugs should include which of the following?
   A. They produce excellent analgesic and antiinflammatory effects but little antipyretic effect.
   B. Antiinflammatory effect occurs immediately after beginning therapy.
   C. Because there is a narrow margin between effective and toxic dosage, levels need to be monitored regularly until therapeutic dosage is established.
   D. all of the above

33. Which of the following is the MOST appropriate nursing intervention to promote adequate joint function in the child with juvenile rheumatoid arthritis?
   A. Incorporate therapeutic exercises in play activities.
   B. Provide heat to affected joints by use of tub baths.
   C. Provide written information for all treatments ordered.
   D. Explore and develop activities in which the child can succeed.

34. An expected outcome for the nursing diagnosis of high risk for body image disturbance related to disease process of juvenile arthritis is:
   A. patient/family are able to explain disease process.
   B. patient is accepted by peers.
   C. patient will express feelings and concerns.
   D. child will understand and use effective communication techniques.

❖ *Crossword Puzzle* ❖

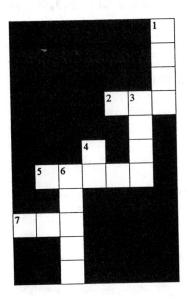

Across

2. Systemic lupus erythematosus
5. Nonsteroidal antiinflammatory drugs
7. Juvenile rheumatoid arthritis

Down

1. Slipped femoral capital epiphysis
3. Legg-Calvé-Perthes disease
4. Juvenile arthritis
6. Slower-acting antirheumatic drugs

❖ CHAPTER 40
The Child with Neuromuscular Dysfunction

1. Identify the following statements as either TRUE or FALSE.

   _____ Upper motor neuron lesions produce weakness associated with spasticity, increased deep tendon reflexes, and abnormal superficial reflexes.

   _____ The primary disorder of lower motor neuron dysfunction is cerebral palsy.

   _____ Lower motor neuron lesions interrupt the reflex arc, causing weakness and atrophy of the skeletal muscles involved, with associated hypotonia or flaccidity with final progression to varying degrees of contracture.

   _____ Lower motor neuron involvement is most often asymmetric.

   _____ In most instances the sudden appearance of flaccid paralysis in a previously healthy child can be attributed to an infectious process.

   _____ Hereditary factors and metabolic disease are more often responsible for muscular weakness and atrophy of gradual onset.

   _____ The most useful classification of neuromuscular disorders defines the source of the lesion: cerebral cortex, anterior horn cells of the spinal cord, peripheral nerves, myoneural junction, and muscle.

2. Match the diagnostic tool with its description.

   A. electromyogram   _____   elevated in skeletal muscle disease; most specific test

   B. nerve conduction velocity   _____   present in skeletal and heart muscle

   C. muscle biopsy   _____   ketamine is used to decrease the pain with this procedure

   D. CPK   _____   measures electric impulse conduction along motor nerves

   E. aldolase   _____   measures electric potential of individual muscle

3. The nurse should know that the etiology of cerebral palsy is MOST commonly related to which one of the following?
   A. existing prenatal brain abnormalities
   B. maternal asphyxia
   C. childhood meningitis
   D. preeclampsia

4. Match the type of spastic cerebral palsy with its description.

A. hemiparesis   _____   pure cerebral paraplegia of lower extremities

B. quadriparesis   _____   involving three extremities

C. diplegia   _____   involving only one extremity

D. monoplegia   _____   similar parts of both sides of the body involved

E. triplegia   _____   most common form of spastic cerebral palsy; motor deficit usually greater in upper extremity; one side of the body affected

F. paraplegia

                            _____   cortical sensory function impairment and therefore impaired two-point

G. parietal lobe syndrome   discrimination and position sense

                            _____   all four extremities equally affected

5. Johnny is suspected of having cerebral palsy because he has clinical manifestations of wide-based gait and rapid repetitive movements of the upper extremities when he reaches for an object. Based on this information, the clinical classification of cerebral palsy Johnny might have is:
   A. spastic.
   B. dyskinetic.
   C. ataxic.
   D. mixed-type.

6. Children with cerebral palsy often have clinical manifestations including alterations of muscle tone. Which one of the following is an example of a child with altered muscle tone?
   A. increased or decreased resistance to passive movements
   B. development of hand dominance by the age of 5 months
   C. asymmetric crawl
   D. When placed in a prone position, the child will maintain the hips higher than the trunk with the legs and arms flexed or drawn under the body.

7. Associated disabilities and problems related to the child with cerebral palsy include which one of the following?
   A. All children with cerebral palsy will have intelligence testing in the abnormal range.
   B. There are a large number of eye cataracts associated with these children which will need surgical correction.
   C. Seizures are a common occurrence among children with athetosis and diplegia.
   D. Coughing and choking, especially while eating, predispose these children to aspiration.

8. The nurse is completing a physical examination on 6-month-old Brian. Which one of the following would be an abnormal finding suggestive of cerebral palsy?
   A. Brian is able to hold onto the nurse's hands while being pulled to a sitting position.
   B. Brian has no Moro reflex.
   C. Brian has no tonic neck reflex.
   D. Brian has an obligatory tonic neck reflex.

9. The goal of therapeutic management for the child with cerebral palsy is:
   A. assisting with motor control of voluntary muscle.
   B. maximizing the capabilities of the child.
   C. delaying the development of sensory deprivation.
   D. surgical correction of deformities.

10. The disease inherited only as an autosomal recessive trait and characterized by progressive weakness and wasting of skeletal muscles caused by degeneration of anterior horn cells is:
    A. Werdnig-Hoffmann disease.
    B. cerebral palsy.
    C. Kugelberg-Welander disease.
    D. Guillain-Barré syndrome.

11. Nursing considerations for the infant with Werdnig-Hoffmann disease should include which one of the following for normal growth and development?
    A. feeding by nasogastric tube
    B. use of an infant walker to develop muscle strength
    C. verbal, tactile, and auditory stimulation
    D. encouraging the parents to seek genetic counseling

12. Diagnostic evaluation for the patient with Guillain-Barré syndrome would include which one of the following results?
    A. elevated CBC
    B. cerebrospinal fluid high in protein
    C. cerebrospinal fluid high in glucose
    D. elevated CPK

13. The priority nursing consideration for the child in the acute phase of Guillain-Barré syndrome is which one of the following?
    A. careful observation for difficulty in swallowing and respiratory involvement
    B. prevention of contractures
    C. prevention of bowel and bladder complications
    D. prevention of sensory impairment

14. Maria, age 5, was born in a South American country and has been in the United States less than one year. While outside playing in the garden, she suffers a minor cut. Since Maria's mother does not think that Maria has ever received immunizations, which one of the following actions would be MOST appropriate at this time to prevent tetanus?
    A. Have Maria go to the clinic tomorrow for the start of administration of all of her needed immunizations.
    B. Administer tetanus immune globulin now.
    C. Administer first injection of tetanus toxoid now.
    D. Administer both tetanus immune globulin and tetanus toxoid now.

15. Nursing implementations for the child with tetanus include:
    A. control or eliminate stimulation from sound, light, and touch.
    B. observe for location and extent of muscle spasms.
    C. arrange for the child not to be left alone, since these children are mentally alert.
    D. all of the above.

16. Infant botulism usually presents with symptoms of:
    A. diarrhea and vomiting.
    B. constipation and generalized weakness.
    C. high fever and decrease in spontaneous movement.
    D. failure to thrive.

17. Nursing considerations for the pediatric patient with botulism include:
    A. teaching the parents the importance of administering enemas and cathartics for bowel function.
    B. preparing the parents for the fact the child will have muscular disability after the illness.
    C. using honey as a formula sweetener to increase oral intake.
    D. teaching parents that boiling is not an adequate prevention.

18. Tammy, age 13, is diagnosed with myasthenia gravis. The nurse, in preparing a teaching plan for the family, includes which one of the following as a priority?
    A. watching for signs of overmedication of anticholinesterase drugs, which include respiratory weakness, choking, and aspiration
    B. encouraging strenuous activity
    C. suggesting to Tammy and her parents to limit Tammy's scholastic accomplishments in school in order to allow for adequate rest
    D. reducing Tammy's weight to reduce symptom occurrence

19. Spinal cord injury causes three stages of response. The second stage is characterized by which one of the following?
    A. spinal shock syndrome
    B. loss of temperature and vasomotor control
    C. replacement of flaccid paralysis by spinal reflex activity which results in spastic paralysis
    D. development of scoliosis

20. Diagnostic evaluation of the child who presents with a spinal injury includes a complete neurologic examination. Motor system evaluation is done by:
    A. stimulating peripheral receptors by eliciting the reflexes like the patellar.
    B. observation of gait and noting balance maintenance.
    C. testing all 12 cranial nerves.
    D. using the blunt end and the sharp point of a safety pin to test each dermatome.

21. Management during the first stage of spinal cord injury may include:
    A. steroid administration within the first eight hours.
    B. ventilatory assistance.
    C. skeletal traction.
    D. all of the above.

22. Children with neurogenic bladder should be taught:
    A. to keep urine alkaline.
    B. how to perform the Credé maneuver to express urine.
    C. that the bladder that empties periodically by reflex action will not need intermittent catheterization.
    D. the necessity of oral antimicrobials administered prophylactically.

23. Clinical manifestations of dermatomyositis include:
    1. proximal limb and trunk muscle weakness.
    2. stiff and sore muscles.
    3. decreased muscle strength and reflex response.
    4. red, indurated skin lesions over the malar areas and nose.
    5. skin over extensor muscle surfaces is erythematous, scaly, and atopic.
    A. 1, 2, and 3
    B. 1, 2, 4, and 5
    C. 3, 4, and 5
    D. 2, 3, and 4

24. Match the major muscular dystrophy with its characteristics. (Dystrophies may be used more than once.)

A. pseudohypertrophic (Duchenne)

B. limb-girdle

C. facioscapulohumeral (Landouzy-Dejerine)

_____ lack of facial mobility; forward shoulder slope

_____ weakness of proximal muscles of both pelvic and shoulder girdles

_____ lordosis, waddling gait, difficulty in rising from floor and climbing stairs

_____ onset in late childhood; autosomal recessive

_____ very slow progression and may have periods with no progression

_____ onset from ages 1 to 3 years

25. Major goals in the nursing care of children with muscular dystrophy include which one of the following?
    A. promoting strenuous activity and exercise
    B. promoting large caloric intake
    C. preventing respiratory tract infection
    D. preventing mental retardation

26. Diagnostic evaluation of muscular dystrophy includes serum levels of CPK, aldolase, and SGOT. When there is severe muscle wasting and incapacitation related to the disease process, the nurse would expect these serum levels to be:
    A. elevated.
    B. decreased.
    C. normal.
    D. unable to accurately be determined with muscle wasting and incapacitation.

❖ Critical Thinking ❖
Case Study

Kenny, age 4, has a history of premature delivery with cerebral palsy being diagnosed shortly after birth. Assessment findings include quadriplegia and deficient verbal communication skills but apparently normal levels of intelligence. Kenny has been hospitalized several times in the past because of respiratory infection and gastric reflux. During Kenny's regular follow-up visit, his mother tells the nurse it is becoming harder to care for Kenny because of his needs. Because of Kenny's recent admission to the hospital for pneumonia, she worries that she is not giving Kenny the care he needs.

27. The nurse should explain to Kenny's mother that one of the complications associated with cerebral palsy is respiratory problems. Which one of the following assessment findings could MOST help explain why Kenny is having these problems?
    A. Kenny has constant drooling, which contributes to wet clothing and chilling.
    B. dietary imbalance with poor nutritional intake
    C. the presence of nystagmus and amblyopia
    D. coughing and choking, especially while eating, and history of gastric reflux

28. Kenny's mother asks the nurse how she can improve Kenny's communication skills, and a diagnosis of impaired verbal communication is developed. Which one of the following plans would be MOST appropriate for Kenny at this time to improve his communication skills?

A. Purchase an electric typewriter or computer to facilitate communication skills.

B. Enlist the services of a speech therapist.

C. Teach Kenny the use of nonverbal communication skills like sign language.

D. Use audio tapes with Kenny to improve his speech abilities.

29. The nurse recognizes that an additional diagnosis is altered family processes related to a child with a lifelong disability. Which of the following implementations should the nurse recognize as being important to include in the plan of care?

A. Explore potential for additional caregiving support.

B. Refer the family to a support group of other parents of children with cerebral palsy.

C. Refer parents to social services for additional suggestions.

D. all of the above

30. Based on the information given about Kenny, what would the nurse expect the MOST appropriate goal for Kenny to be?

A. Kenny will acquire mobility.

B. Kenny will acquire self-help abilities and care for his basic needs.

C. Kenny will increase his ability to communicate.

D. all of the above

❖ Crossword Puzzle ❖

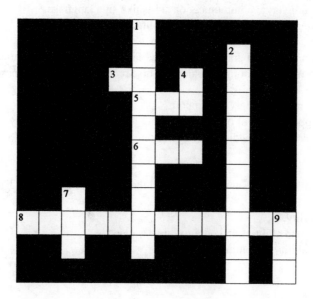

Across

3. Cerebral palsy
5. Electromyogram
6. Tetanus immune globulin
8. Paralysis of all four extremities

Down

1. Increased muscle tension
2. Paralysis of lower extremities
4. Myasthenia gravis
7. Tetanus antitoxin
9. Activities of daily living

❖ ANSWERS
Page References

CHAPTER 1

1. p. 3
2. p. 4
3. p. 4
4. p. 4
5. p. 5
6. p. 5
7. p. 6
8. p. 6
9. p. 6
10. p. 7
11. p. 7
12. p. 7
13. p. 7
14. p. 7
15. p. 8
16. pp. 11-12
17. p. 11
18. p. 11
19. pp. 12-13
20. pp. 13-14
21. p. 15
22. pp. 15-16
23. p. 16
24. pp. 17-22
25. p. 22
26. p. 23
27. p. 24
28. p. 24
29. p. 24
30. p. 24

CHAPTER 2

1. p. 29
2. p. 30
3. p. 31
4. pp. 32-37
5. p. 38
6. p. 38
7. p. 38
8. p. 38
9. p. 38
10. p. 39
11. p. 39
12. p. 39

13. p. 40
14. p. 40
15. p. 40
16. pp. 40-41
17. p. 41
18. p. 42
19. pp. 41-44
20. p. 44
21. p. 45
22. pp. 45-46
23. p. 45
24. pp. 47-48
25. p. 49
26. p. 48
27. p. 49
28. p. 50
29. p. 55
30. p. 55
31. p. 56
32. p. 45
33. pp. 45-47 and 51-55
34. pp. 56-60

CHAPTER 3

1. p. 66
2. pp. 66-70
3. pp. 70-71
4. p. 72
5. p. 75
6. pp. 75-76
7. p. 76
8. p. 76
9. p. 77
10. p. 78
11. pp. 79-80
12. p. 80
13. p. 82
14. p. 81
15. p. 82
16. p. 84
17. p. 85
18. p. 86
19. p. 86
20. p. 87
21. p. 91
22. p. 94

34. p. 1466

CHAPTER 34

1. p. 1494
2. p. 1494
3. p. 1495
4. p. 1495
5. p. 1495
6. p. 1498
7. p. 1498
8. p. 1498
9. p. 1498
10. p. 1500
11. p. 1501
12. p. 1501
13. pp. 1502-1503
14. p. 1503
15. pp. 1505-1506
16. p. 1507
17. p. 1507
18. p. 1507
19. p. 1507
20. p. 1508
21. p. 1508
22. p. 1514
23. p. 1512
24. p. 1512
25. p. 1516
26. p. 1517
27. pp. 1518-1519
28. p. 1530
29. pp. 1519-1529
30. p. 1520
31. pp. 1526-1529
32. pp. 1519-1529
33. pp. 1519-1529
34. p. 1530
35. p. 1531
36. p. 1531
37. p. 1531
38. p. 1532
39. p. 1532
40. p. 1533
41. p. 1533
42. p. 1533
43. p. 1533
44. p. 1533
45. p. 1534
46. p. 1534
47. p. 1534
48. p. 1535
49. pp. 1534-1535
50. pp. 1534-1535
51. p. 1535
52. p. 1535

53. pp. 1535-1537
54. p. 1537
55. p. 1540
56. pp. 1540-1541
57. p. 1541
58. p. 1542
59. p. 1543
60. p. 1543
61. p. 1545
62. p. 1545
63. p. 1545
64. p. 1546
65. p. 1547
66. p. 1548
67. p. 1549
68. p. 1550
69. p. 1552
70. p. 1553
71. p. 1556
72. p. 1529
73. p. 1538
74. p. 1538

CHAPTER 35

1. pp. 1564, 1565, 1566, and 1568
2. p. 1567
3. p. 1569
4. p. 1569
5. p. 1607
6. pp. 1572 and 1576
7. p. 1573
8. p. 1577
9. p. 1578
10. p. 1577
11. p. 1578
12. p. 1579
13. p. 1579
14. p. 1580
15. p. 1580
16. p. 1582
17. p. 1583
18. p. 1585
19. p. 1589
20. p. 1592
21. p. 1592
22. pp. 1593-1594
23. p. 1595
24. p. 1595
25. p. 1597
26. p. 1597
27. p. 1598
28. p. 1599
29. p. 1601
30. pp. 1602-1603
31. pp. 1604-1605

12. p. 1747
13. p. 1748
14. p. 1750
15. p. 1752
16. p. 1753
17. p. 1754
18. p. 1754
19. p. 1756
20. p. 1757
21. p. 1758
22. p. 1761
23. p. 1763
24. p. 1763
25. pp. 1764-1765
26. pp. 1765-1766
27. p. 1768
28. p. 1770
29. p. 1771
30. p. 1772-1773
31. p. 1776
32. p. 1779
33. p. 1781
34. pp. 1783-1784
35. p. 1785
36. p. 1765
37. p. 1786
38. p. 1787
39. p. 1787

CHAPTER 39

1. p. 1795
2. p. 1798
3. p. 1804
4. p. 1808
5. p. 1806
6. p. 1809
7. p. 1817
8. p. 1816
9. pp. 1812-1814
10. p. 1819
11. p. 1822
12. p. 1823
13. p. 1827
14. pp. 1824-1826
15. pp. 1830-1831
16. p. 1832
17. p. 1835
18. p. 1837
19. pp. 1838-1841
20. p. 1844
21. p. 1844
22. p. 1845
23. pp. 1846-1847
24. pp. 1847-1848
25. p. 1848

26. p. 1850
27. p. 1854
28. p. 1856
29. p. 1862
30. p. 1864
31. p. 1858
32. p. 1858
33. p. 1862
34. p. 1862

CHAPTER 40

1. pp. 1869-1870
2. p. 1871
3. p. 1871
4. p. 1872
5. p. 1872
6. p. 1873
7. p. 1873
8. p. 1874
9. p. 1874
10. p. 1882
11. p. 1884
12. p. 1884
13. p. 1885
14. p. 1886
15. p. 1887
16. p. 1887
17. p. 1888
18. p. 1888
19. p. 1892
20. p. 1893
21. p. 1895
22. p. 1896
23. p. 1899
24. p. 1899
25. p. 1901
26. p. 1902
27. p. 1873
28. p. 1880
29. p. 1879
30. p. 1878